"This is your guidebook to the road ahead."

Every physician who believes in a better-informed patient should read *Information Therapy*. This breakthrough book reinvents the concept of information prescriptions and suggests how clinicians should be paid for writing them.

Albert G. Mulley Jr., MD, MPP
Chief, General Medicine Division, Massachusetts General Hospital
Author and editor of *Primary Care Medicine*

Information Therapy is a must-read book for anyone who cares for patients—or has ever been sick. It's no secret that traditional methods of patient education are hopelessly ineffective. The book's proposal to *reimburse* clinicians for *prescribing* information is brilliant!

Susan Edgman Levitan
President, The Picker Institute

Information Therapy builds a new bridge between patient education and the practice of medicine. Sensible, doable, enlivened with patient stories, *Information Therapy* updates and reinvigorates patient education.

David S. Sobel, MD, MPH
Director, Patient Education and Health Promotion, Kaiser Permanente Northern California
Coauthor of *The Healthy Mind, Healthy Body Handbook*

Calling upon years of Healthwise wisdom, along with their hallmark humor and plain style, Don Kemper and Molly Mettler have created a superb introduction and guide to the new world of patient health care coproduction.

Richard G. Rockefeller, MD
President, Health Commons Institute

Information Therapy brings new focus to the importance of shared decision making and patient-centered care. This concept is a key part of reengineering the future of health care.

George B. Bennett
Chairman and CEO, Health Dialog

Patients who are actively engaged in their own care do better than those who are not. Don Kemper and Molly Mettler are longtime leaders in the development of effective, understandable information for patients. This book synthesizes their wisdom and advances the information therapy agenda.

Margaret E. O'Kane
President, National Committee for Quality Assurance

Information Therapy gives us a new perspective and a new vocabulary for improving health and well-being. The role of information therapy will increase in the future. This is your guidebook to the road ahead.

Ian Morrison, PhD
Author of *The Second Curve: Managing the Velocity of Change*

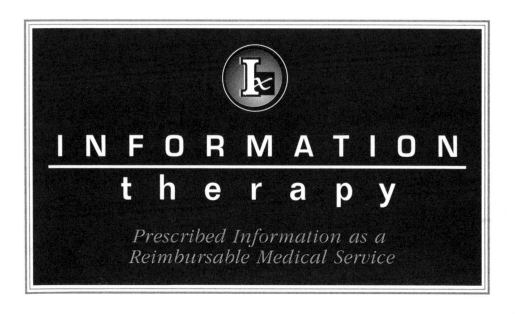

INFORMATION therapy

Prescribed Information as a Reimbursable Medical Service

Donald W. Kemper, MSIE, MPH

Molly Mettler, MSW

Center for Information Therapy,
a division of Healthwise, Incorporated

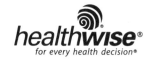

healthwise®
for every health decision®

Cover design by Jamie Lloyd and text design by Terrie Britton

Information Therapy: Prescribed Information as a Reimbursable Medical Service
First Edition, 2002

Ix^{TM} is a trademark of Healthwise, Incorporated.

Prescription-Strength Information^{TM} is a trademark of Healthwise, Incorporated.

Healthwise, Healthwise Knowledgebase, and the Healthwise logo are trademarks of Healthwise, Incorporated, registered in the U.S. Patent and Trademark Office. Other publications of Healthwise, Incorporated, include *Healthwise*® *Handbook, Healthwise*® *for Life*, and *Salud en casa: Guía práctica de Healthwise*®. All other names and logos are (registered) trademarks of their respective holders.

This book and other Healthwise publications are available at special discounts for bulk purchase. Please contact Healthwise, Incorporated, at 1-800-706-9646, or visit our Web site at www.healthwise.org.

ISBN 1-877930-88-1

Printed in the United States of America

Printed on recycled paper

Reader: Please also visit www.informationtherapy.org.

Table of Contents

Acknowledgements

Information Therapy is a book of suggestions and proposals itching to take action. The fundamental ideas that form the heart of the book have been nurtured, scrutinized, and hotly debated by scores of smart people. We are especially indebted to Vernon Wilson for his simple statement all those years ago, "The consumer is the greatest untapped resource in health care"; C. West Churchman and Henrik Blum of UC Berkeley for insights into the purpose and meaning of the health care system and the consumer's role within it; David Sobel for a decades-long friendship and for clear thinking on patient-centered care; Al Mulley and Jack Wennberg for sculpting the concept of shared decision making into an evidence-based science; Tom Ferguson for always, always, emphasizing how important the consumer's role truly is; and David Bradley, Rushika Fernandopulle, and Pranav Kothari for taking bold steps in applying information therapy concepts within hospitals.

Every person on the Healthwise staff has contributed, in ways large and small, to the book's creation. We appreciate working with such a fine group of professionals. We are especially indebted to the gracious Katy Magee, our primary (and patient!) editor; Steve Schneider, Healthwise's chief medical officer, for his clinical guidance and review of the patient stories; Jo-Ann Kachigian, Terrie Britton, John Kubisiak, and Andrea Blum for copy editing, layout, and production management; Gene Drabinski, Josh Seidman, and Bob Long for substantive help in moving information therapy ideas from concept to reality; Mary Ellen Lemon, Annette Phillipp, Sarah Bosarge, and Michelle Vicars for answering many pesky research questions; Phyllis Royston and Michelle Wood for setting up www.informationtherapy.org; and Brenda Foster and Karen Baker for careful reviews and suggestions for improvements.

We also thank the founding members of the Information Therapy Commission for their faith that information therapy will fundamentally change health care:

Susan Edgman-Levitan	James L. Field
Albert G. Mulley Jr., MD, MPP	Annette O'Connor, PhD, RN
Margaret E. O'Kane	Peter J. Plantes, MD
John Rother	John W. Rowe, MD
Edward Wagner, MD	Paul Wallace, MD

This book is dedicated to our treasured mothers, Barbara Mettler and Dorothy Kemper, who taught us that it's important to try to make a difference in the world.

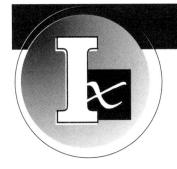

Information therapy, the radical idea that people should have access to accurate, evidence-based information as part of their treatment, is an important and visionary advance in medical care.
David M. Lawrence, MD, MPH

Information Therapy

Information is medicine—powerful medicine. Information is as important to a patient's health as any drug, medical test, or surgery. When the right information is prescribed to the right person at the right time, it becomes "information therapy."

Most patients greatly value the information and advice they receive from their physicians. Yet the way doctors and patients exchange information is generally inefficient, incomplete, and outmoded. With new information technologies, physicians, clinics, hospitals, and health plans can now reinvent patient education to match the needs and demands of today's consumer. By offering every patient the right information prescription as part of the process of care, the health care system can achieve measurable improvements in medical outcomes, patient safety, the overall cost-effectiveness of care, and patient satisfaction. New clinical and business applications built on information therapy (Ix) concepts are already providing significant advantages that physicians, hospitals, clinics, and health plans need in order to thrive.

What Is Information Therapy?

- **The right information**: Evidence-based, approved by experts, up to date, and referenced

- **The right person**: The patient or caregivers who will share in the decision or behavior change

- **The right time**: Just in time to help make a better medical decision or to improve a health behavior

Information can be prescribed, just like a pill. It can come in different strengths, different dosages, and different formulations. When information is personalized and directed to a specific patient at just the right time to help the patient make a specific health decision, the information's value increases exponentially.

Prescription-Strength Information

Not all information is created equal. To be considered "prescription-strength" and worthy of information therapy, information should meet seven essential criteria:

1. **Decision-focused:** Helps achieve better decisions.

2. **Evidence-based:** Uses a balanced review of all relevant research

3. **Reviewed by experts:** Approved by clinicians in each relevant specialty of medicine

4. **Referenced:** Identifies authors and sources

5. **Up to date:** Revised on a regular basis to keep pace with medical advances

6. **Free from commercial bias:** Developed and presented objectively

7. **User-friendly:** Presented in a form and language that patients can easily understand

To meet the work flow requirements of clinical practice, Prescription-Strength Information must also be "intelligent." Intelligent content is indexed to billing codes and structured medical languages so that relevant information options can be instantaneously presented to the physician or patient as an integrated part of the care process.

Three Ways to Prescribe Information Therapy

Physician-Prescribed Information Therapy

The most potent information prescriptions are made directly by the physician based on the physician's knowledge of the patient and what medical decisions he or she faces. All physicians do this now, but without the benefit of technology support, training, or reimbursement incentives. With support from handheld computers, information prescriptions will become an important part of every physician visit.

System-Prescribed Information Therapy

System-prescribed information therapy occurs when health information systems automatically "push" targeted information (using "standing orders") to a patient by e-mail, phone, or fax based on what the system already knows about the patient's decision-making needs. When delivered correctly, system-prescribed information will revolutionize shared decision making. System-prescribed information can be automatically sent with every medical lab report, medication prescription, and preauthorization notice.

Consumer-Prescribed Information Therapy

There is no stopping the consumer's quest for medical information—nor should there be. In the new medical era, the patient is a full partner with the physician on the "provider" team. As a member of the team, patients should have as much access to medical information about themselves and their condition as they want to have, without restriction and without a professional's prescription.

For consumers untrained in medical research, however, prescription-strength content must be made available through systems that are easy to search and understand. Self-prescribed or consumer-prescribed information connects the patient with the information either through direct searches or by referral from self-help groups, family members, or friends.

Seven Opportunities for Information Therapy

Health care decisions and behavior can be influenced at every point along the health care continuum from prevention and wellness to chronic disease management and end-of-life care.

In each of the following opportunities, getting the right information to the right patient at the right time can significantly benefit both the patient and the health care system.

1. **Prevention.** Routine information prescriptions can greatly extend the preventive services reach of most medical centers from the limited set of immunizations and screenings they now do to a full array of ongoing support in the areas of fitness, nutrition, stress management, and safety.

2. **Self-care.** Self-care is what a person does to recognize, prevent, treat, and manage health problems on his or her own. Information prescriptions, whether self-prescribed or otherwise, help people do these things better.

3. **Self-triage.** Self-triage decisions focus on a few key decision steps in seeking medical care: Should I go? When should I go? Where should I go? And how should I go? Getting the right information to the patient in time to help with these decisions can save both lives and dollars.

4. **Visit preparation.** A well-prepared patient gains much greater value within the time constraints of a brief office visit. Previsit information prescriptions that help the patient prepare for and anticipate what will happen in the visit will lead directly to better decisions, better outcomes, and more satisfied patients. Such visit-prep information prescriptions can become standard procedure for virtually all medical visits through the use of computerized scheduling systems.

5. **Self-management of chronic illnesses.** For many chronic diseases like diabetes, arthritis, and hypertension, successful treatment depends on daily adherence to healthy self-management behaviors. Regular information prescriptions to both patients and caregivers can provide valuable and timely encouragement to support adherence to jointly developed self-management plans.

6. **Decision support.** Of the seven areas of significant opportunities for information therapy, the one that may offer the greatest potential benefit is that of decision support. In the near future, no major decision for a drug, surgery, or invasive medical test will likely be done without information prescriptions to help the patient participate in the decision.

7. **End-of-life care.** Prescribing information to patients and caregivers as a part of end-of-life care has both huge potential and complex challenges. Emotionally sensitive communication of the right information at the right time can help guide families toward decisions that will best meet their needs through the patient's final days of life.

Information Therapy as a Safety Net

Patients who are at high risk for medical errors often feel vulnerable and powerless to protect themselves. In spite of the best efforts of their doctors, nurses, and hospitals, thousands of Americans are harmed by medical mistakes each year. Information prescriptions received at the hospital bedside can help a patient or caregiver monitor medications, anticipate procedures, and prepare for the next step in the care process. With the right information prescriptions, the patient and caregivers can provide an additional level of protection against medical errors.

Prescription Information as a Reimbursable Medical Service

One reason that the methods and quality of communication between doctor and patient have not kept pace with other advances in medicine stands out: nobody pays for it. In most cases, a doctor who takes the time to explain treatment options and solicit informed preference information from the patient gets the same reimbursement as one who does not. Three things have blocked the reimbursement of patient education in the past: unverifiable quality, uncertain clinical appropriateness, and documentation difficulties. New Ix technologies can overcome each of these barriers. Prescriptions of evidence-based decision-support information "written" by a physician at the time a diagnosed patient is considering treatment options will eventually be covered as part of the reimbursement formulas.

Opportunities for a Rebirth of E-Health

Information therapy is powerful enough to breathe new life into scores of e-health business plans that have foundered. First-generation "content" business plans were based on the flawed idea that information had value in and of itself. Early content sites were akin to giving the patient a key to the pharmacy but not helping him or her to know when to go, what to look for, where to look, or what dose of medicine to take. The results were unpredictable and, far too often, of little value. Information therapy adds value by connecting the right information to the decision making that influences medical outcomes and medical costs.

Predictions for an Information Therapy Future

We're making three predictions for the next decade:

- Every clinic visit, lab test, prescription drug, or treatment will result in a targeted information prescription to the patient.

- Every hospital admission and every change in hospital-based physician orders will result in a targeted information prescription for the patient.

- Information prescriptions will be built into the reimbursement formulas for clinic and hospital visits.

Information therapy is the defining strategy that transforms medical care into patient-centered care. It redefines the role of the patient as a full partner in medical decision making and as a bona fide member of the provider team. And information therapy redefines the role of information from being *about* care to being a basic *part* of care. The right information delivered to the right person at the right time is powerful medicine.

The best way to predict the future is to invent it.
Alan Kay

1

The Case for Information Therapy

Let us tell you a true story about a 40-something woman we know very well. We'll call her Ms. M.

Ms. M, an enthusiastic if inept skier, ended up in a hospital emergency room one winter weekend with very pronounced knee pain. What happened in subsequent weeks is a fairly typical story of patient bewilderment, conflicting opinions from multiple doctors, and disjointed follow-up care. We'll tell you what transpired and how much better it could have been for everyone if Ms. M, in addition to the standard remedies, had been prescribed **information therapy: the right information at the right time.**

The moral of the story is this: Information is powerful medicine. Correctly prescribed information is as important to a patient's health as any drug, medical test, or surgery.

Woman Goes to a Doctor . . .

Here's how the story goes: Ms. M hurts her knee skiing and goes to an emergency room where she gets some X-rays. The ER doctor splints the knee and advises her to see her primary care physician. The ER nurse gives Ms. M a blurry handout on how to care for her hurting knee at home.

The next day, her primary care doctor refers Ms. M to an orthopedic specialist. When she is able to get an appointment 3 days later, the specialist looks at the X-rays, does a physical exam, and then diagnoses a torn ACL (anterior cruciate ligament). Torn ACLs are a very common knee injury and often the toll extracted for going too fast on icy slopes. The specialist, who has treated many a torn ACL, recommends reconstructive surgery. He does not explain, however, the surgery's risks or benefits, nor does he suggest any alternatives. Stalling for time, Ms. M writes down the name of the procedure so she can do some research on her own. At home, Ms. M does her own Internet search on "torn ACL" and finds an array of information—some good, some weird. She decides to seek a second opinion.

Orthopedic specialist No. 2 confirms the diagnosis but recommends a different reconstructive surgery, saying that the first recommended surgery isn't as effective for a person of Ms. M's . . . er . . . advanced years. Ms. M is baffled by the options: what should she do? In truth, she wants to avoid surgery. Specialist No. 2 orders an MRI to assess the extent of knee damage. He also orders a bone density test for chronologically gifted Ms. M. The radiology results come back in "radiologic-ese," that is, not understandable to Ms. M. The specialist must interpret the results for Ms. M, who learns from the tests that she has an alternative to surgery—intensive physical therapy, which she quickly opts for. She also learns that her bone density is less than optimal. Uh-oh. Osteopenia. Ms. M gets referred to a physical therapist for follow-up care for her knee injury. However, Ms. M gets no advice or information on follow-up care for her weakening bones.

Six weeks elapse from accident to first PT session, time in which Ms. M could have begun to do some simple rehab exercises on her own, saved some sweat and tears about what to do, and gotten a lot smarter about her health. At every point in this process, Ms. M would have greatly benefited from "information therapy."

This simple book is all about delivering information therapy—the right information to the right person at the right time—in hopes that Ms. M and millions of people like her can participate with their doctors in getting better health care.

Information Therapy (Ix) Defined

The quick definition of right information, right person, right time tells most of the Ix story. A more formal definition is also useful:

> Information therapy is the prescription of specific, evidence-based medical information to a specific patient, caregiver, or consumer at just the right time to help them make a specific health decision or behavior change.

The Right Information

To make a difference, information should be decision-focused and evidence-based. If information doesn't help make better decisions, it doesn't really help.

Consumers have access to health information on the Internet that is mostly accurate, but too general to be of particular help. Consumers also have access to information that is wildly, dangerously inaccurate ("21-day cancer cures," "electronic zappers for brainworms," . . . No, we are not making this up). For information to be therapeutic, it must be accurate, evidence-based, up to date, and unbiased. And it must delve deeply enough to address the specific clinical concerns that challenge the patient.

To be truly therapeutic, information must be strong enough to qualify as "prescription-strength." It must make a difference in the life and care of the patient.

The Right Person

To make a difference, information must reach the people who will make and support the decision.

The right person is the person or people directly involved in making a specific health decision or

Information therapy is the prescription of specific, evidence-based medical information to a specific patient, caregiver, or consumer at just the right time to help them make a specific health decision or behavior change.

changing a specific health behavior. The right person can be the patient alone, or the patient with a spouse, a family member, a close friend, or any other invited advocate. Each health care professional who is part of the provider team may also be considered one of the right people to receive the information.

The Right Time

To make a difference, information must be available at the time of the decision or the needed action.

The right time is "just in time" to make a health decision. Presented too early, the information may go unused and forgotten. Presented after the decision is made, it is usually too late. For maximum effectiveness, the information must be presented during the time all options are being considered.

The concept of information as therapy is ancient. Medical advice has always been at the heart of medicine. Doctors and patients agree that the most valuable of all medical services is the advice given by physician to patient. Information therapy intensifies that value.

But information therapy will also revolutionize health care. As information is redefined as a true therapy, its quality standards, availability, and effectiveness must also be redefined. When the patient is added to the provider team, the information tools used by the patient must be brought up to the same quality level as the tools used by the rest of the team. Once this informed and well-equipped patient becomes the norm, the entire practice of medicine will take an evolutionary—and revolutionary—leap.

The Patient Is on the Provider Team

You have probably heard the phrase "patient as provider." Some people have been talking for decades about self-care, shared decision making, and patient-centered care. Clearly, patients do provide care for themselves and their families. What is subtly different here is recognizing that self-care and shared decision making are not just important for the patient but essential to the health care system itself. The patient is not just a part of the system; the patient, as the primary care provider, is at the center of the system. You can't have "patient-centered care" without the patient.

To the contrary, however, health professionals have been taught both in school and in practice that patients and providers are on different sides of the fence. Health professionals provide care to patients; patients receive the care. The distinction used to work just fine. Not so anymore. The "new consumer" wants information, choice, and service as a part of the health care experience. And those requests are not frivolous. Informed and engaged in their own care, most patients can help their doctors better focus treatment plans on their needs, better accomplish the recovery goals they set, and more often avoid the medical mistakes that might otherwise cause death or disability.

Putting patients on the team can be a very good thing, but it does require a little adjustment. When you think of the patient as an equal member of the provider team, three things become necessary: the patient must have the same access to information that other team members have; the patient's information and actions must be well connected with those of the other team members; and the patient must succeed for the team to succeed.

If none of this sounds overly profound, stick with us. Treating the patient as a respected member of the team is the key to finding success in this new era of care.

Information Is Care

Health information is not just *about* care. Information *is* care. It is as important to care as a medication, a lab test, or a surgical procedure. Information guides patient decisions and changes patient behaviors. With good information, patients can often heal themselves. Without it, they can do themselves harm, overlook effective cures, and undermine the best-laid clinical plans.

Again, the shift from information being about care to information as care is small and easy to dismiss. Don't dismiss it. When information is seen as care, it triggers new standards of quality and new expectations. It also becomes a reimbursable service. As laid out in Chapter 8, three barriers have stood in the way of reimbursement for information prescriptions: information quality, documentation requirements, and appropriateness. Information therapy removes those barriers and opens the way for introducing information prescriptions into reimbursement formulas.

Invent the Future:
Prescribing Information

Consumers are providers of care, but the scope of their focus differs from that of professional providers. Consumers generally focus on one patient only—themselves. They care about one diagnosis only—their own. They want to know one main thing—what they should do next.

Prescribing information is the perfect strategy to tap into that focus. An information prescription uses existing information about the patient to anticipate the health decisions he or she will be facing. It pinpoints information that will help that patient reach the best decision and delivers the information just in time to help that patient make the decision. And information prescriptions can provide documentation for everyone on the care team: the patient, the doctors and nurses, and others.

Prescribing information has some compelling advantages over the Internet search engine method most people now use to find health information. Those advantages include:

- **Convenience.** The information is prescribed for and delivered to the patient. The patient spends zero time hunting for information. This convenience can greatly increase the number of patients using good information.

- **Quality.** Prescribed information from a verified source can be certified to be evidence-based, up to date, and unbiased.

- **Integration.** Because prescribed information is delivered within the health care system, physicians, nurses, or other professionals can directly refer to it. Information can also be automatically customized to match the health situation and demographics of the individual.

Prescribed information also has a distinct advantage over traditional methods of doctor-patient communication in its ability to maximize the value of that information. For most people, the traditional doctor-patient exchange results in patients neither getting all the information they need nor retaining the information they do get.

Consider this scenario: Out of all the useful information available to help with a particular decision, an average physician on an average day probably remembers about half of it. During a typical office visit, however, the physician has the time to tell the patient only about two-thirds of what he or she remembers. The patient hears and understands correctly only a portion of that information and remembers an even smaller portion once he or she leaves the doctor's office. After these successive losses of information, most patients get home with only a small fraction of the information that could help them with the health care decisions they are facing.

Information prescriptions in combination with traditional doctor-patient communication can stop a lot of the information decay. An information prescription delivered to the patient can clearly present all of the most valuable points. In addition, applying multimedia and learning theory methods to the presentation of the information can boost patient understanding. Heavy reliance on the patient's memory is also eliminated because the information can be reviewed again at home.

Delivering Information Therapy

While information therapy happens any time the right information is delivered to the right person at the right time, it can be categorized into three general types based on how and by whom it is prescribed.

Physician-Prescribed Information Therapy

The exchange of information between an individual and his or her physician is the most valued service in medicine. People trust their doctors for

---

Ix Delivery

1. *Physicians can prescribe it.*

2. *Health systems can prescribe it.*

3. *Consumers and self-help groups can prescribe it.*

---

information and advice to help them decide what they should do to prevent, cure, or live with health problems. For many patients, when information comes from a physician, it has extra value. When it comes from a physician who knows and has examined the patient, it has even greater value.

Because people trust their doctors, the most potent information prescriptions are those made directly by a person's physician. Physicians and other clinicians add value in two direct ways. First, by selecting the information that they think the patient most needs, they help the patient focus on the key issues. Without that, the patient may have a very difficult time pulling useful information from reams of printouts or scores of Web pages in related, but not specifically helpful, areas. Second, by prescribing information to patients, physicians change the patients' expectations about their role. Often that is the only invitation that patients need to become engaged. Without the invitation, they are not sure if their involvement is welcome. With it, they begin to feel like members of the team.

It's getting easier for clinicians to prescribe information. With the introduction of handheld computers for order entry, medication prescriptions, and electronic medical records, clinicians have a tool for making information prescriptions a part of every clinical encounter.

The widespread adoption of physician-prescribed information therapy will integrate the new role of the patient and the new role of information into the practice of medicine. Through it will come the very best in patient-centered care as it strengthens the role of the physician and makes the doctor-patient relationship even more robust.

Physician-prescribed information will not be enough, however. If the goal is to connect the right person with the right information at the right time, limiting information prescriptions to the clinician-patient exchange only will cause us to fall short of the goal. Why? Some decisions are made before the patient has any contact with the physician, and frankly, many physicians will be slow to adopt both information technology and information therapy into their practices. We need to think systemwide.

System-Prescribed Information Therapy

Enormous investments in information technology have been made by hospitals, clinics, and health plans over the past decade. These improvements in information infrastructure provide a strong foundation for enhancing the reach and value of information prescriptions. System-prescribed information therapy occurs when health information systems automatically "prescribe" targeted information to a patient by e-mail, secure messaging, phone, or fax based on the physician's standing orders and information the system has recorded about the patient's decision-making needs.

Frankly, information prescriptions from a faceless "system" will never be as potent as those prescribed directly by the patient's doctor. A professional with knowledge of the patient can quickly scan the most likely information prescriptions and select the one that best matches the patient's needs. With the professional involved, the information prescription can drill down to a very specific level and literally say to the patient, "Read this and call me in the morning." That may indeed be the gold standard. With system-prescribed information, the patient must narrow down the information. The system can generate a selection of information prescriptions, each of possible value, but patients must select from those the prescriptions that make the most sense for them.

Even with that limitation, however, the value of system-prescribed information therapy is considerable. With the right technology in place, system-prescribed information can be sent automatically with every medical lab report, medication prescription, or preauthorization notice. System-prescribed reminders are already being credited with improvements in immunization rates and increased participation in health screenings. When delivered correctly, system-prescribed information will revolutionize shared decision making within the practice of medicine.

Consumer-Prescribed Information Therapy

Information therapy in no way implies that access to information can be limited "by doctor's prescription only." Quite the contrary— information therapy can be self-prescribed or provided by a person's family, friends, or anyone else to whom the patient turns. In the new era of medicine, the patient is a full partner with the physician on the provider team.

Self-prescribed or consumer-prescribed information therapy connects the patient with the right information either through direct searches on the Internet or by referral from others. Concerned family members are highly motivated to help their loved ones find good information. They can develop and send consumer-prescribed information at virtually no cost by e-mail. Self-help groups are another case in point. While their work goes largely unrecognized in professional health care, self-help groups help millions of people make health care decisions every day. These groups can use Ix prescriptions to standardize what information they provide and how they provide it.

Three Families

To illustrate the practical application of information therapy without compromising patient privacy, we have created three families for use throughout this book. The stories of three American families—the Morrisons, the Gomezes, and the Williamses—are referred to in subsequent chapters to demonstrate how prescribed information improves health care. Each family is based partly on reality (each medical situation is a true one) and partly on fiction (we have burdened each family with more than their fair share of health problems).

The Morrison family

Mary Morrison, 46, suffers from chronic sinusitis and toenail fungus. She also has occasional heartburn. Her husband, Jack Morrison, 49, gets his cholesterol tested. Daughter Susan, 12, hurts her wrist in a basketball game. Grandmother Lori Nelson, 73, is considering a hip replacement.

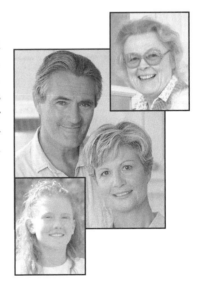

The Gomez family

Alicia Gomez, 31, hurts her knee (tearing her anterior cruciate ligament) playing pick-up soccer. Her son, Billy, 6, has behavioral and learning differences that concern Alicia but are as yet undiagnosed.

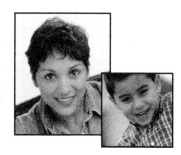

The Williams family

Jackson Williams, 59, suffers from urinary problems because of an enlarged prostate. He is also a long-term smoker. His daughter, Jane, 30, goes to see her doctor because she's fatigued and feeling "out of sorts."

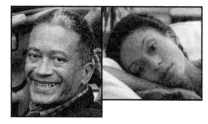

Information therapy has value only if it can help people like the Morrisons, the Gomezes, and the Williamses better manage their health problems. Information therapy is for real people living in the real world. These stories will speak for themselves.

Toto, I have a feeling that we're not in Kansas anymore.
Dorothy

2

Four Drivers of Health Care Change

The Chinese ideogram for crisis combines two words: "danger" and "opportunity." Literally translated, crisis means "opportunity riding the dangerous wind."

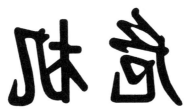

Crisis: Opportunity Riding the Dangerous Wind

These days, the words "health care" and "crisis" seem permanently wedded. No one would contest that we're in the middle of a health care quandary. The *dangers* are well known to us: systems failures in cost, access, and quality, critical staffing shortages, the aging of the population . . . The list goes on and on. Yet there are *opportunities* embedded in the current crisis—opportunities that, if recognized, embraced, and managed, could drive the fundamental reshaping of the American health care delivery system. These drivers are the rise of the new consumer, the rise of evidence-based medicine, the rise of the Internet, and the focus on quality and accountability. Separate, yet interrelated, these four drivers are shaping the future roles of patients and physicians and the delivery of care. They truly are opportunities riding the dangerous wind.

We're Different: The New Consumer

We're knowledgeable, we're demanding, and we're the new majority. Study after study heralds the emergence of the "new medical consumers," those Americans with the college education, the cash, the computer experience, and the heightened expectations to make significant demands upon the health care system of the twenty-first century. In her book *Market-Driven Health Care*, Harvard professor Regina Herzlinger summed up what today's consumers want: convenience and mastery.[1]

Heralded by the first wave of Baby Boomers, the ranks of the new consumer will make up about half of the U.S. population by 2005.[2] Already, the purchasing patterns and habits of the new consumer have transformed many U.S. retail and service industries. Finance, travel, and other retail services are available, buffet-style, for the informed and savvy consumer to select among. Health care has lagged behind these other industries, but it seems very likely that the new medical consumer's expectations and preferences will have a demonstrable impact on health care delivery.

According to a report from the Institute for the Future, the new consumers are a different population altogether from those who came before:[3]

- **We're more sophisticated when it comes to making health care choices.** The new consumers have had more years of education. With even just one year of college course work behind them, the new consumers make their choices—about a doctor, a health plan, or a treatment—more analytically than those who have had no college training. Analytical decision making tends to lead to comparative choices, which has a direct impact on health care spending because . . .

- **We've got money to spend.** The new consumers have enough disposable income not to be limited to the least expensive health care options. This financial flexibility lets the new consumers apply their analytical skills in health care decisions. It also encourages consumers to look farther and wider for information and follow through with their decisions. This is easier for the new consumers because . . .

- **We know our way around a computer.** The new consumers have more experience with information technologies such as computers and the Internet because they use them at work and home. The Internet, of course, opens up access to information previously beyond the reach of all but the most dedicated health information seekers.

Taken together, analytical methods, disposable income, and greater access to information are creating a class of health care consumers that is unprecedented in its makeup and behavior.

Consumer expectations have changed too. Research gathered from consumer focus groups reveals that:[4]

- **The consumer is taking charge.** Empowerment is evident in all levels of consumer participation in health care.

- **Consumers are redefining choice.** They are willing to change doctors, institutions, and health plans. They are also seeking choice in treatment and care options.

- **Consumers, particularly Baby Boomer women, are gathering lots of information about their health** from both traditional and nontraditional sources. They expect to be able to use that information when making health care decisions.

These expectations underscore a profound change in just where the center of health care sits. Expectations of choice, control, and, particularly, information require shifting the consumer's role from that of *patient* to *partner*.

We already see that shift in the move by hospitals and health plans to "patient-centered care" and "consumer-centric care." Patient-centered care refers to the partnership between the physician and the patient regarding health care and the various choices involved in treatment and healing. Patient-centered care holds that a physician cannot and should not attempt to make critical decisions regarding choices among various treatment options without first understanding what the patient wants. Hospitals and other health care organizations tout their patient-centered care as a means of attracting new patients and increasing patient satisfaction and loyalty. Consumers go looking for it, believing that they have the right to the full quality of life they desire

Surgeries With Widest Variation

The following surgeries show the greatest variation in rates across the 306 hospital regions studied:

1. *Partial mastectomy*

2. *Prostate removal*

3. *Angioplasty*

4. *Lower extremity revascularization*

5. *Carotid endarterectomy*

6. *Back surgery*

7. *Thigh fracture repair*

8. *Hip replacement*

9. *Leg amputation*

10. *Heart valve replacement*

Statistics from *The Dartmouth Atlas of Health Care, 1999,* reported in *USA Today.*[5]

and that only they know precisely what is right for them. Whatever the perspective, with these heightened expectations, and with the majority of the U.S. population easily fitting into this new defining class, the new consumers will have an indelible impact on the way health care is delivered.

We're Getting More Knowledgeable: The New Science of Evidence-Based Medicine

Is medicine an art or a science? Physicians pride themselves on the intuition they develop for diagnosing health problems and selecting the treatment that best fits their patients' needs. Based on apprentice-like learning from their training and their medical mentors, and reinforced by observations from their own clinical experience, physicians develop unique styles of practice. Applied this way, medicine is an art.

When medicine is largely practiced as an art, certain peculiarities emerge. One result of highly individualized patterns of practice is that a population of patients with the same health problem can receive widely differing treatments and achieve widely varying outcomes. Suffer from low back pain in Harlingen, Texas, and you have a 1.5 percent chance that the problem will be addressed with surgery. Take that same low back pain to Santa Barbara, California, and your chances for surgery go up over 300 percent. People in Lancaster, Pennsylvania, are 3.3 times as likely to receive cardiac catheterization as people in Grand Junction, Colorado. Men in Billings, Montana, are 8 times as likely to have radical surgery for enlarged prostate as men in Tuscaloosa,

Alabama. Variations like this aren't even transcontinental; they can occur within a region. A male resident of Fort Worth, Texas, is almost twice as likely to get a radical prostatectomy as a man living in Houston. Conversely, there is 58 percent more surgery for cardiac catherization in Houston than in Fort Worth. The list goes on and on, and it's simply not logical.[6]

These variations in clinical practice are tracked and reported in *The Dartmouth Atlas of Health Care*,[7] and they reveal an unsettling truth: in medicine, geography is destiny. The treatment you receive is more dependent on where you live and which physician you see than on what the science says or what you personally prefer. The differences in surgical rates across the country "illustrate a surgical environment for patients filled with what *Atlas* researchers call uninformed consent. It is a situation, they say, born of inadequate medical science, opinion parading as knowledge, over-reliance on inadequately verified diagnostic tools, and basic inequities in the health care system."[8]

Scarily enough, a lot of what happens to you in health care is based solely upon the opinion of the physician treating you. However, a new model for medical practice is emerging—one in which the *science* of medicine is emphasized. The new discipline of evidence-based medicine de-emphasizes intuition, small-sample or anecdotal observations, and the common practice of other local physicians as the primary basis for medical decision making. According to the authors of *Evidence-Based Medicine*:

> Evidence-based medicine (EBM) is the integration of best research evidence with clinical expertise and patient values. . . . When these three elements are integrated, clinicians and patients form a diagnostic and therapeutic alliance which optimizes clinical outcomes and quality.[9]

Painstaking research on the outcomes of medical treatments and interventions is leading to the construction of practice guidelines and clinical pathways that result in the best health outcomes for the most patients. Slowly but surely, evidence-based medicine is making headway—and it needs to. For example, it is known that treatment with beta-blockers after a person suffers a heart attack reduces the chance of a subsequent attack between 20 and 30 percent. However, many cardiologists have been slow to routinely prescribe them. Managed care

Medical Guidance Systems

Clinical guidelines have been criticized as a one-size-fits-all approach to medical care. Dr. Richard Rockefeller of Health Commons Institute (HCI) promotes "medical guidance" systems as a physician- and patient-friendly alternative. Medical guidance forgoes rigid guidelines in favor of a system that allows physician and patient "to go wherever we wish safely and reliably, with maximum leeway for variable human preference and idiosyncrasy." HCI says that getting to medical guidance requires:

- *Computer-based clinical decision-support tools.*

- *Communication systems that facilitate doctor-patient partnerships and integrate health care into an efficient, scientific enterprise.*

- *Human systems that can adapt to new technologies and changing health care needs.*

To learn more, go to www.healthcommons.org.

❖

plans with practice guidelines and a way to measure their implementation have substantially increased beta-blocker use for their members. In just one year (1999-2000), the percent of heart attack patients who were not prescribed beta-blockers decreased 29 percent, from 15 percent to 10.7 percent.[10]

Art Meets Science

Following the dictates of outcomes research, health plans, hospitals, and physician groups are spending millions of dollars to encourage their doctors to accept practice guidelines. Some physicians have been slow to adopt new guidelines, especially when they see the guidelines as conflicting with the art of medicine. If they cannot use their education, experience, and judgment to decide how they practice medicine, some physicians will reject efforts to force them into guidelines, no matter how good the science may be. The challenge is to transform the art of medicine into something that is more compatible with the new science—something that allows physicians to use their education, experience, and judgment to apply evidence-based guidelines to the special needs, values, and preferences of each patient.

For art to meet science, three things need to be in place: physician expertise, evidence-based practice guidelines, and informed patients. These three things can be vastly aided by information technology that brings the best medicine to physician and patient alike.

We're Wired: The Internet

Until recently it was almost impossible for patients to get medical information relevant to their needs. Few medical libraries were open to the layperson, and few public libraries had professional medical tomes in their stacks. Medical information meted out by physicians to patients in the clinic was limited to handouts and the occasional brochure. Hospital patients were lucky to get anything at all. Too frequently, the patient was left in the dark about his or her health situation and had to depend solely on what the doctor remembered to convey.

The Internet has changed all that. (And how!) There are reportedly about 52 million adult Americans—55 percent of the online adult population—using the Internet for reasons related to health care. Nearly half of these health information seekers said that the online material influenced their decisions about treatment.[11] Forever gone are the days when the average patient had to struggle to get beyond the basics.

Many, many Americans are finding just what they need on the Internet, but danger lurks out there. What has replaced the reality of the uninformed patient is the specter of the wrongly informed patient.

The Wild, Wild Web

What the Internet does not lack is abundant information. What the Internet does lack is quality control over the information that is there, the way that it is organized, and how people can access it. Let's tackle the quality of the information first, focusing on the most flagrant example of poor quality: Internet quackery.

Type in "arthritis" in a Web search (or "hair loss" or "allergy" or any other health issue that is troubling you), and you'll have a sporting chance that some of the information you get back will be simply wrong, fraudulently wrong, or criminally wrong.

Internet quackery preys upon the all-too-human desire to be thinner, healthier, pain-free, and just plain alive. And con artists stand to make a lot of money by promising those results. Take, for example, these Internet opportunities:

- Exercise while lying down. A $660 device will give you "all the cardiovascular benefits of a workout without the spine-jarring effect of running or jogging." Lie flat on your back while the machine replicates "the undulation of the spine based on the way fish swim and four-legged mammals walk, . . . a uniquely stress-free yet highly aerobic form of exercise."[12]

- If undulating sounds like too much work, you can always order a device that uses "far infrared rays" in "maintaining general health and also helping to prevent various diseases. . . . If you have been suffering from chronic ailments for a long time, give this a try! See for yourself if it can't restore YOUR lost vitality. Enjoy thermo-therapy while you sculpt the figure you've always wanted. Feel ter-rific, too!" Yours for just $899.00 plus tax and shipping.[13]

- You can't go wrong with multipurpose remedies. "See what Dr. Moss wrote about the coffee enema at *Coffee: The Royal Flush.* . . . Please browse through our site to find out more about the products we offer as well to purchase them on-line. We offer a range of . . . fountain syringes for taking the occasional enema and Colema® boards for irrigating your colon. *We also have great organic coffee for drinking as well as cleansing.* [Italics ours.]"[14]

At a minimum, taking up the offers of these health care "helpers" is guaranteed to set a consumer back by hundreds of dollars. Consumers also run the risk of forgoing evidence-based treatment for very real problems and avoiding the dull, boring, sensible stuff (eat less, exercise more) that is the foundation of good health. But in the main, these are relatively harmless suggestions . . . well, except perhaps for the coffee enemas.

However, the health Internet also blithely offers up information that is frighteningly, recklessly erroneous. Consider these promises:

- A cure for HIV/AIDS guaranteed to work in 5 days. Note that this cure is predicated upon the following "medical facts": "The human intestinal fluke *(Fasciolopsis buskii)* is the source of the HIV virus. This parasite typically lives in the intestine where it might do little harm, causing only colitis, Crohn's disease, or irritable bowel syndrome, or perhaps nothing at all. . . . If it establishes itself in the thymus, it causes HIV/AIDS! AIDS is a condition. When the thymus gland cannot "make" enough T cells, your immunity is lowered. Benzene is the cause of AIDS." The purported cure is designed to kill the parasites.[15]

- A cure for cancer. The "New 21 Day Program for Advanced Cancers" cure package can be yours for only $1782.78. "Caution: It is intended for severely ill patients and not for prevention purposes."[16]

- A cure for depression. From an article entitled "ADD-ADHD Depression Cure" found on the Web: "All persons I have seen with clinical depression had small roundworms in the brain. . . . If you suffer from depression use your zapper to immediately kill these four roundworm species: *Ancylostoma*, *Ascaris*, *Trichinella* and *Strongyloides*. Other family members should be cleared of these four worms on the same day or as close to it as possible. Re-infection always occurs. In the depressed person, the microscopic parasites travel immediately to the brain. In others, they may simply reside in the intestine or lungs or liver, or other organs. Pathways (routes) to the brain have become established for the depressed person. These must heal before there is any tolerance for re-infection." You, the consumer, can zap away your depression with the "New Super Zapper DeLuxe." $149.00 plus tax and shipping.[17]

Granted, these are extreme examples of erroneous health information. But even a systematic survey of 25 reputable Web sites indicated that health information on the Internet is "inefficient, incomplete and incomprehensible."[18]

The California HealthCare Foundation commissioned RAND Health to look at Web-based information, in both English and Spanish, on four conditions: childhood asthma, breast cancer, depression, and obesity. A panel of physicians judged whether or not the information contained all of the clinical elements they thought important to cover. As reported in the *Journal of the American Medical Association* in May 2001, there is good news—the "accuracy of the information provided is generally good."[19] But there's not-so-good news too:

- **Health information on the Web is often incomplete.** For example, only 1 in 5 English-language sites provided complete and accurate information about managing the initial symptoms of a severe asthma episode. Spanish-language sites were more likely to suffer from incomplete information.

- **Many sites contradict themselves.** For example, one childhood asthma site stated in one place that inhaled steroids do not stunt growth and then reported in another that they do stunt growth. (FYI: Some inhaled steroids taken in large doses do delay growth in some children.)[20]

- **Search engines, the most often used tools for finding health information on the Web, may be the weakest link.** Consumers using English-language search engines had a 1 in 5 chance of finding relevant information on the first page of results; with Spanish-language engines, consumers had only a 1 in 9 chance of finding relevant material.

- **Web-based information currently demands a high degree of health literacy.** All of the English-language sites had material that required at least a tenth-grade reading level; more than half had material presented at the college level. (The "new consumers" may be college-educated analytical thinkers, but most of them aren't health professionals. When medical information has a high reading level, fewer people will be able to understand it—period.)

Yes, the quality of health information on the Internet is highly inconsistent. And, yes, the options for the consumer are mind-boggling. However, the capability of the Internet to deliver information is proven. It is indeed a powerful resource that has changed the landscape of American health care. For laypeople, the challenge lies in obtaining and interpreting credible, unbiased, consumer-focused, evidence-based information so that they can participate with their physicians in making medical decisions. Health plans and others Internet providers have discovered their Web sites serve more than a marketing role. Increasingly frustrated in their efforts to sort through dense and often conflicting information on the Web, Internet users now flock to personal and proprietary sites in an effort to find quality information.

Consumers are clamoring for a place at the table, and information technology is pulling out the chair for them.

We're Aware:
The Focus on Quality and Accountability

For decades health care professionals have been trying to patch together a highly fragmented system (think total quality management and continuous quality improvement), but efforts to implement quality improvement processes were largely unnoticed and unreported except by a few on the fringe. No one owned the problem. But then, in 1999, the Institute of Medicine (IOM) published a report that brought the problem to real public attention. *To Err is Human* blasted into the headlines with the alarming news that 44,000 to 98,000 Americans die every year because of medical mistakes.[21] Hearing that, the public woke up . . . and shuddered.

What is especially worrisome is that the thousands upon thousands of medical errors cited by the report were those found in hospital cases, yet hospital patients represent only a small percentage of the total population that is intersecting with the health care system. Patients are seen in outpatient surgical centers, physician offices, and clinics. Patients are cared for in homes and in institutional settings such as nursing homes. Patients go to retail pharmacies to have prescriptions filled. Medical errors can occur in these settings as readily as in a hospital. We are all vulnerable.

The response to this initial report was swift and loud. Health plan associations called for mandatory reporting of medical errors. The White House supported the development of a patient-safety center. Consumer groups called for improved hospital quality and better reporting of mistakes. Continuing medical education programs and quality monitoring programs all got an extra jolt of "quality fever." By pointing out the urgent problem of patient safety, the report succeeded in focusing public and media attention on quality issues in health care.

To Err is Human was but the first shot across the bow. The IOM, along with other groups such as the Institute for Healthcare Improvement, continues its Herculean efforts to make quality the foundation for lasting and positive change in the health care system. It isn't going to be easy. The IOM's 2001 report, *Crossing the Quality Chasm*, begins with the observation:

"*Our challenges are not marginal and their solutions are not incremental.*"

Donald Berwick, MD,
Institute for Healthcare
Improvement

❖

The American health care delivery system is in need of fundamental change.... Quality problems are everywhere, affecting many patients. Between the health care we have and the care we could have lies not just a gap, but a chasm.[22]

Bridging chasms requires not only strong structural engineering but also the initial leap of faith. Implementing major and dramatic changes in how health care is delivered is no small task. Donald Berwick, MD, president and CEO of the Institute for Healthcare Improvement, has said that, "Our challenges are not marginal and their solutions are not incremental."[23] The call for quality improvement in health care is nothing short of a call for revolution.

As health care professionals working within a system sorely in need of radical change, we need to be asking ourselves a number of questions:

• What will it take to fully embrace the new consumer and expand the role of the consumer into all aspects of medical care?

• What will it take to broaden the reach of evidence-based medicine to physicians as well as consumers? What might be the impact in terms of quality, costs, and satisfaction if all consumers, regardless of their insurance coverage, had access to the best evidence-based consumer health information to help them in all aspects of their medical decision making, be it self-care for common problems or complete shared decision making for major and chronic health problems?

• What will it take to step up and insist on discipline within the Internet? Without a focus on quality control, the current health Internet is as likely to bring the *wrong* information to the right person at the right time as it is to bring the right information.

- What will it take to recognize that any effort to build quality and patient safety requires the full involvement of the consumer and the need to build systems for that consumer involvement?

In *Crossing the Quality Chasm*, the IOM recommends ten simple rules to guide the design of a revolutionized system that is more responsive to patients. The rules are printed in their entirety in the Notes on pages 229 and 230.[24] Let us draw your attention to the first five rules. They clearly highlight the need for information therapy—the right information to the right person at the right time.

1. **Care based on continuous healing relationships.** Patients should receive care whenever they need it and in many forms, not just face-to-face visits. This rule implies that the health care system should be responsive at all times (24 hours a day, every day) and that access to care should be provided over the Internet, by telephone, and by other means in addition to face-to-face visits.

2. **Customization based on patient needs and values**. The system of care should be designed to meet the most common types of needs, but have the capability to respond to individual patient choices and preferences.

3. **The patient as the source of control**. Patients should be given the necessary information and the opportunity to exercise the degree of control they choose over health care decisions that affect them. The health system should be able to accommodate differences in patient preferences and encourage shared decision making.

4. **Shared knowledge and the free flow of information**. Patients should have unfettered access to their own medical information and to clinical knowledge. Clinicians and patients should communicate effectively and share information.

5. **Evidence-based decision making**. Patients should receive care based on the best available scientific knowledge. Care should not vary illogically from clinician to clinician or from place to place.

There is a role for information therapy in the coming health care revolution. The four drivers of health care change—the new consumer, the trend toward evidence-based medicine, the rise of the Internet, and the demand for quality and accountability—all call for a new way to engage the patient at the center of care. They all call for getting the right information to the right person at the right time. They all call for information therapy.

Caveat emptor. (Let the buyer beware.)
Ancient Roman consumer advocate

3

Prescribing Information

There's the right kind of information to prescribe and the right time to prescribe it. This chapter looks at both.

The Right Kind: Prescription-Strength Information

Not all health information makes the grade for information therapy. As you've seen in Chapter 2, there's plenty of information available to consumers that is plain wrong, weirdly wrong, or dangerously wrong. There's also information that is too weak and too shallow to truly inform and guide the patient. And, saints preserve us, there's information that has the taint of commercial bias.

You'll want to ask some basic questions about the information that you are considering as the foundation for your information therapy efforts:

- Who is compiling the information?

- Where is it coming from?

- Who stands to gain from the information that is shared?

- Will consumers be able to understand the information?

- Will four out of five doctors recommend it?

Criteria for Prescription-Strength Information

1. *Decision-focused*

2. *Evidence-based*

3. *Reviewed by experts*

4. *Referenced*

5. *Up to date*

6. *Free from commercial bias*

7. *User-friendly*

Information has to be strong enough to make a difference in the life of the patient and trustworthy enough to be accepted by practicing physicians. For information therapy to work, the information offered must be **prescription-strength**.

To be considered prescription-strength, to indeed be the "right" information for the patient, information should meet seven essential criteria. It must be decision-focused; evidence-based; reviewed by experts; referenced; up to date; free from commercial bias; and consumer-friendly.

1. Decision-Focused: Does It Really Help?

If information doesn't help people make better decisions, it doesn't help. This message is so critical to the success of information therapy that it bears repeating: **If information doesn't help people make better decisions, it doesn't help.**

Information prescriptions can be focused around three types of decisions: direct medical care decisions, health behavior decisions, and quality control decisions.

Direct Medical Care Decisions

Direct medical care decisions are directly related to the questions people face as they move through an illness or health condition. They involve questions like: Are these symptoms serious? Should I see a doctor now, today, or later? Do I need this medication? Do I need this proposed medical test? Do I need this proposed medical treatment?

Inherent within each question is a decision that the patient and physician must usually make together. Sometimes the decision is straightforward and easy to make—"Yup, my arm is broken, better get it set." Other decisions can be complex and difficult to make.

When the decisions are complex, the patient is oftentimes left with having to go in search of the needed information. Perhaps the search leads to a medical encyclopedia, or a health Web site, or a brochure. Accurate, up-to-date medical encyclopedias may have all the correct information, but if they do not focus on medical decisions, they will have limited value for the patient. Their information is not prescription-strength.

Consider the lowly bunion. For the interested and bunion-afflicted consumer, it just takes a modem, a mouse, and a moment to gain access to about 7,000 Web sites connected to bunion information. A random trawling of the information can yield very basic bunion surgery information ("Surgery is recommended to correct the deformity, reconstruct the bones and joint, and restore normal, pain-free function"),[1] alternatives to bunion surgery ("Magnetic Insoles: Massage and Relieve Sore, Achy Feet Fast"),[2] and detailed scientific articles about aspects of bunion surgery ("Hallux Valgus: Pre- and Postoperative Radiographic Evaluation").[3]

To arrive at a *decision* about what to do about his or her particular bunion, the consumer has to sort through this welter of information or simply rely on the advice of a physician.

Having a focus on decisions makes the information more personal, more useful. General information on medical conditions and medical treatments is certainly helpful as background material, but general information, no matter how deep and finely crafted, does not provide the patient-centered "they're talking about me!" message that targeted, specific information prescriptions can supply.

Make the information decision-focused, and patients get what they need. Decision-focused Prescription-Strength Information lays out not only descriptive information about bunions but also home treatment for bunions, when surgery is indicated, what different kinds of surgery are available, the risks and benefits of each surgical approach, the outcomes of the surgery (Can the bunion come back? Are people generally satisfied with the results?), other treatment options, questions to ask the doctor and surgeon, and an opportunity to think through personal values and preferences.

Whether they are for bunions or breast surgery, information prescriptions need to clearly identify content that helps bring important decision-related information into focus for the consumer. Only information prescriptions that help improve decisions about medical care reach the full status of being therapeutic.

Health Behavior Decisions

Health behavior decisions are choices and actions a person makes that will affect his or her health. There are actions a person can take to prevent illness and promote overall health and well-being. A person can quit smoking, start exercising, start flossing . . . or not. The opportunity is there. And, for every chronic condition, there are actions that a person can take to increase his or her ability to manage the disease. With diabetes, for example, a patient can take action (or not) on diet and nutrition, on home blood sugar monitoring, on foot care, and on knowing what to do in case of a diabetic emergency.

How can information itself change the tendency to choose the "or not" option? By being action-specific. Decision-focused action plans can help consumers focus on unambiguous, achievable, and manageable things to do. Action plans can provide action-oriented tools and information that consumers can use in the day-to-day management of their health conditions. They can contain information that helps people better understand the effect of the actions they take. Action plans can also include interactive quizzes and assessments for people to measure their knowledge. The ultimate purpose of this type of behavior-focused information is to help the individual develop, begin, maintain, and experience positive health behavior success.

Quality Control Decisions

Decision-focused information therapy can also provide valuable support with "quality control decisions." Here the benefit comes in the ability of the information to help people determine if they are getting the *level of quality care* that they are seeking. For example, a previsit information prescription can encourage a diabetic patient to expect a foot examination at every visit. If, in the rush of a clinical encounter, the physician forgets the exam, it is easy for the patient to correct the error right then, right on the spot.

2. Evidence-Based: Is It True?

The drive toward evidence-based medicine is fueled by two truths: 1) there is too much information for any one individual to access and use; and 2) health care practice is not always based on good evidence. Once again in health care, we have a situation in which more is not necessarily better.

There *is* too much information. Medical information is growing in such scope and complexity that physicians are finding it increasingly difficult to stay current:

> . . . (There are) about 20 clinical journals in adult internal medicine that report studies of direct importance to clinical practice. . . . To keep up, the dedicated doctor would need to read about 17 articles a day every day of the year.[4]

These dozen-plus articles, even if read, don't begin to cover the clinical practice information that also appears in subspecialty journals, clinical economics studies, and marketing materials from various vendors. Policy developers and managed

---

A Patient's Action Plan for Type 1 Diabetes

- *Dealing with negative feelings about the diet for diabetes*
- *Using a "plate format"*
- *Using a food guide for diabetes*
- *Counting carbohydrates*
- *Monitoring your blood sugar at home*
- *Preparing and giving an insulin shot*
- *Caring for your feet*
- *Caring for your eyes*
- *Dealing with low blood sugar level emergencies when you take insulin*
- *Preventing high blood sugar emergencies*

---

care are also weighing in with an ever-expanding compendium of clinical guidelines, profiling, and utilization review.

It's not enough to just read the stuff. In addition to sorting out which abstracts and articles to read, today's clinician must also determine if the evidence presented is good evidence, if the new ideas for diagnosis, treatment, and predicting outcome actually do work.

> Most busy doctors lack the time or skill to track down and evaluate this evidence. . . . Many cannot keep up. Consequently, there is a widening chasm between what we ought to do and what we actually do.[5]

The need to know what actually works—how to mine the gems from the mountains of information—has given rise to *evidence-based medicine* (EBM). EBM endeavors to cross the chasm between "what we ought to do and what we actually do."

Evidence-based medicine is the process of finding, reviewing, and using research findings as the basis for clinical decisions.[6] Several organizations have come to the fore to facilitate this collection process, among them the Cochrane Collaboration (www.cochrane.org), an international not-for-profit research organization that aims to help people make informed decisions about health care,[7] and the U.S. Department of Health and Human Services' Agency for Healthcare Research and Quality (www.ahrq.gov).[8]

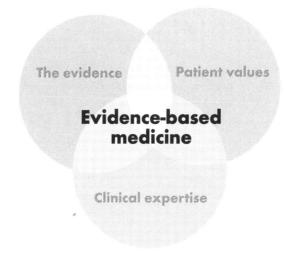

Advocates are quick to add that EBM is not "cookbook" medicine. Instead, as David Sackett and his colleagues note in *Evidence-Based Medicine*, it is the integration of three things: the best research evidence, clinical expertise, and patient values.[9]

The *evidence* refers to clinically relevant research drawn from all relevant human, animal, and laboratory research. There are hierarchies of the quality of the evidence, as illustrated in Table 3.1.

The *individual clinical expertise* of the physician is needed to decide whether the external evidence is applicable to the individual patient and how that evidence should be incorporated into a clinical decision. Data from a group of patients in a study cannot match the patient perfectly; clinical expertise is needed to bridge the gap.[10]

Table 3.1 Quality of Evidence

I: Evidence obtained from at least one properly randomized controlled trial

II-1: Evidence obtained from well-designed controlled trials without randomization

II-2: Evidence obtained from well-designed cohort or case-control analytic studies, preferably from more than one center or research group

II-3: Evidence obtained from multiple time series with or without the intervention

III: Opinions of respected authorities, based on clinical experience; descriptive studies and case reports; or reports of expert committees

Source: U.S. Preventive Services Task Force, *Guide to Clinical Preventive Services.*[11]

Patient values are those personal preferences, concerns, and expectations that each individual patient brings to the clinical encounter. While two women with early-stage breast cancer may have the same risks and the same information, they may arrive at very different treatment decisions because they weigh the costs and benefits of each treatment from their own unique perspectives.

How Do You Judge Whether the Information Is Evidence-Based?

Developing evidence-based information requires careful research. Content development teams must know how to rate the quality of evidence behind the original information and how to judge whether the quality is high enough to be used within an information prescription. Often in medical care, the documented evidence base is weak, even though there is strong medical opinion in support of a practice or treatment. In such cases Prescription-Strength Information should rely on the best available evidence without overstating the proof behind it.

Content providers must be on the lookout for geographical bias. Research into geographic variations of medical practice clearly points out the influence of local norms over medical science.[12] The writers and reviewers of medical information can be significantly influenced by the practice patterns of the physicians around them. This local practice bias can come into play even in the interpretation of well-done, randomized clinical trials. While much protection is gained by selecting medical writers and reviewers who are trained to look for the "evidence" behind each procedure or practice, further protection against geographic variation can be gained by selecting clinical experts from widely diverse geographic areas to review the content.

Content developers will start with the best evidence, from peer-reviewed journals and clinical guidelines from major health care organizations and other responsible agencies, and interpret it for consumer use so that it is as unbiased as possible.

It must be said that only the thinnest layer of current clinical practice is truly evidence-based. It must also be said that the scope and reach of evidence-based medicine are increasing. Evidence-based medicine is perhaps the single most important vehicle available today for assuring high-quality health care. When combined with a patient's personal preferences and a doctor's experienced judgment, it is the foundation of wise health decisions.

3. Reviewed by Experts: Who Says So?

When judging the quality of information made available to consumers, you'll want to know: Who says so? Can I trust the source?

Expert medical review of Prescription-Strength Information is essential to high-quality information therapy. Yes, skilled medical librarians can identify and rate the evidence on medical research findings. And yes, skilled writers and editors can effectively interpret that information for consumer use. However, for information to be considered prescription-strength, it needs to be reviewed and sanctioned by licensed medical experts.

Expert review provides two primary benefits. First, expert review improves the quality of the content. Practicing specialists can use their training, experience, and judgment to protect the writer and the reader from representations that might mislead or confuse patients in real medical situations. The physician specialist's in-depth knowledge of a medical area allows him or her to review and shape the content from a focused perspective that is beyond the purview of the generalist writer or researcher.

Second, expert review adds to the credibility of the content; information with zero credibility has zero value. For patients and physicians to accept information prescriptions as valuable, they must have reason to believe that the information is medically accurate. The best way to do that is to reveal the credentials of the medical reviewers and to describe the editorial process used to develop the information.

It's not enough to simply have a "medical review board." A requirement for Prescription-Strength Information is to *identify which reviewers examined which sections* of the information. The practice of recruiting a broad board of medical experts but relying on only a few undesignated individuals to review the bulk of the content is misleading.

4. Referenced: Can I Trust the Source?

Referencing of the material is particularly critical. Today's physicians face a difficult challenge in dealing with the patient who walks into the office with an armload of Internet downloads. Within the limited time available during a clinic visit, physicians have no real way to judge the quality of the information other than to quickly eyeball the authors' credentials and the source of the material. Physicians are much more likely to accept medical information that carries the imprimatur of a peer-reviewed journal, such as the *Journal of the American Medical Association* or the *New England Journal of Medicine*, than the medical gems offered up by a glossy women's magazine.

Referenced Prescription-Strength Information identifies who wrote and compiled the information and on what sources the information is based.

5. Up to Date: How Current Is the Information?

Keeping consumer health information fresh can be likened to painting the Golden Gate Bridge: just as soon as the crew gets to the end of the bridge, it's time to start over at the beginning. The same is true for those who update prescribable information. The job is never done.

Want to find prescription-strength content? Look for content providers that have developed a systematic process of review for every piece of information—a tough and daunting task. Prescription-Strength Information needs to be updated when changes in medical practice warrant it. Content providers must react quickly to new research findings that might have a significant impact on medical decisions. Once new findings are reviewed and accepted into the medical knowledge base, there must be a process in place to quickly modify the information that is prescribed to patients.

In addition, once developed, information needs to be reviewed and updated on a regular basis. The update schedule can vary by topic depending on how "active" the research is. Topics that have ongoing research and rapidly changing treatment, such as diabetes, coronary artery disease, and HIV/AIDS, need to be on a frequent update schedule. Topics with relatively stable information—say stress management or treatment for animal bites—may not need to be updated as often.

Alas, keeping current is not as simple as linking a site to a medical news service. There's a delicate balance in finding the right mix of what's current and medically acceptable and what's just "new." Up-to-date information incorporates new medical evidence that has been reviewed and accepted broadly within medical practice. Being current and up to date does not require the inclusion of every newly reported finding. Frequently, it takes time to assess the quality of the research and evaluate how the new findings contribute to the foundation of previously tested and accepted evidence.

Keeping information state of the art also poses major challenges for content providers that attempt to make information available in other languages or for special populations. A one-time translation of information into Spanish or Braille, for instance, has little long-term value without an accompanying commitment to update the translations as the original source of the information is updated.

How will *you* know if the information you are viewing meets the criterion of being up to date? Information that is truly prescription-strength will clearly indicate when it was developed and when it was last reviewed.

6. Free From Commercial Bias: Is It Objective?

We inhabit an economy that celebrates a free market. Naturally, individuals and organizations want you to buy their products and services, and, if they have the means, these folks are going to do their darnedest to convince you that their product is the best available. There's nothing wrong with that, except when it comes to Prescription-Strength Information.

Prescription-Strength Information must be written from a perspective that is focused solely on the patient's best medical, economic, and legal interests. Information that is slanted by the bias of other interests just won't cut it.

The ethical standard for full disclosure of influence on content by commercial sponsors is present in all major ethical codes, including the Hi-Ethics Principles (www.hiethics.org), the URAC Health Web Site Accreditation Program (www.urac.org), the eHealth Code of Ethics (www.ihealthcoalition.org), the Health on the Net (HON) Foundation (www.hon.ch), and the American Medical Association (www.ama-assn.org).

These codes of ethics state that commercial sponsor influence on either the preparation of content or the selection of content must be clearly disclosed to the user. Several of the codes explicitly extend the disclosure requirement to include a description of any sponsorship arrangements that influence the priority listings of search engine results. While the "pay-for-position" approach has been part of many search engines for years without explicit disclosure of the sponsorship relationships, full disclosure is needed to meet the highest ethical standards.

While there is a general ethical requirement for medical information to be free from *undisclosed* commercial bias, information prescriptions should try to go one step further: be free from commercial bias, undisclosed or otherwise. Those who create the information and those who review it should have no significant economic stake in the consumer's choice of medical treatments and services.

The effects of commercial bias are not limited to the creation of the content. Commercial influence on how content is presented or how Web search engines prioritize findings can also steer people inappropriately toward one medical decision over another. While fully disclosed influence over search engines and information presentation is legal and perhaps acceptable in certain sponsored venues, it has no place within the core of Prescription-Strength Information.

Although the concept of a bias-free presentation of information and choices is central to the ethical practice of medicine, there is clearly a significant gap between concept and practice. It is well established that changes in economic incentives change the frequency of surgical procedures and other treatments ordered by physicians. It is also clear that the very companies that will profit from the sale of specific drugs fund much of the research into the effects of those drugs. While the medical world may not be as perfect in these areas as we might like, there is clear opportunity for the information therapy industry to develop a higher standard.

7. User-Friendly: Can It Be Understood?

Just about every piece of medical information comes with two (or more) names: the scientific or technical label that is bandied about by health professionals and lobbed over the heads of most patients—otitis media, benign prostatic hyperplasia, edema—and the everyday translation—ear infection, enlarged prostate, swelling. Patients often complain that medical professionals talk over their heads. For information to be useful to the patient and the patient's family, it needs to be translated from technical terminology into language that is easily and readily understood. Prescribable information, if it is written for the consumer, will help with the translation process.

The definition of user-friendly information goes beyond language. The use of images, sound, animation, and video can help to actively engage consumers in learning more about their health problems and treatment options. With medical information in particular, a picture is truly worth a thousand words. A good mix of multimedia information can take the consumer into the inner workings of the human body, increase consumer understanding of what's really going on, and, hopefully, enhance decision making.

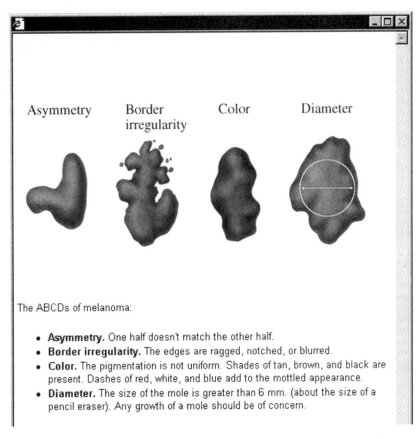

Asymmetry   Border   Color   Diameter
irregularity

The ABCDs of melanoma:

- **Asymmetry.** One half doesn't match the other half.
- **Border irregularity.** The edges are ragged, notched, or blurred.
- **Color.** The pigmentation is not uniform. Shades of tan, brown, and black are present. Dashes of red, white, and blue add to the mottled appearance.
- **Diameter.** The size of the mole is greater than 6 mm. (about the size of a pencil eraser). Any growth of a mole should be of concern.

In Information Therapy, a Picture's Worth a Thousand Words[13]

And Make the Content "Intelligent" Too

In addition to meeting the seven required criteria for Prescription-Strength Information, the best content is also "intelligent." Intelligent content is information whose metadata includes tags, embedded codes, or index tables that link the information to diagnosis, medication, and procedural codes, or to the richly structured medical languages used to extract information from large medical databases.

When information is intelligent, it can be used to "trigger" information prescriptions both with and without the physician's direct involvement. Intelligent tagging can be applied to hundreds of different structured languages, codes, and ordering systems. Four of the most common are discussed in more detail on pages 103 to 105.

The Right Time: Seven Opportunities for Information Therapy

Health care decisions and behavior can be influenced at every point along the health care continuum from prevention and wellness to chronic disease management and end-of-life care. Information prescriptions can be useful at all of these points in the continuum of care.

Prevention

Many clinics and health care systems have developed a method for dispensing routine prevention messages—"Time for your flu shot!" Targeted and personalized information prescriptions can greatly extend that service by offering a full array of ongoing support in the areas of fitness, nutrition, stress management, and safety.

Once established, automated secure messaging systems fueled by specific information about each patient can cost-effectively deliver, document, and update a prevention encouragement and reminder program custom-designed for each individual. (See page 84 for an example of a prevention-oriented information prescription.)

Opportunities for Information Therapy

1. *Prevention*
2. *Self-care*
3. *Self-triage*
4. *Visit preparation*
5. *Self-management of chronic illness*
6. *Decision support*
7. *End-of-life care*

Self-Care

Self-care is what a person does to recognize, prevent, treat, and manage health problems on his or her own. Information prescriptions, whether self-prescribed or otherwise, help people do these things better. (See page 48 for an example of a self-care information prescription.)

Self-Triage

Self-triage decisions focus on three key decision steps in seeking medical care: Should I go? When should I go? Where should I go? Information prescriptions that get the right information to the patient at the time of these decisions can save both lives and dollars. There's another benefit: Improving self-triage may also alleviate nursing shortages in emergency departments by eliminating nonurgent visits. (See page 120 for an example of a self-triage information prescription.)

Visit Preparation

A well-prepared patient is an efficient and effective patient. He or she will gain much greater value within the time constraints of a brief office visit (and quite possibly ease the burden of a busy and harried physician). Previsit information prescriptions that help the patient prepare for and anticipate what will happen in the visit will lead directly to better decisions, better outcomes, and more satisfied patients. Such visit prep information prescriptions could become standard procedure for virtually all medical visits through the use of computerized scheduling systems. (See page 50 for an example of a visit prep information prescription.)

Self-Management of Chronic Illness

For many chronic diseases like diabetes, arthritis, and hypertension, patient adherence to daily self-management behaviors holds the key to success. Regular information prescriptions both to patients and to caregivers can provide valuable and timely encouragement to support adherence to jointly developed self-management plans. (See page 92 for an example of a chronic disease self-management information prescription.)

Decision Support

To have surgery or not? To opt for a lumpectomy or mastectomy? To take the medicine or try the alternative therapy? What decision do I make? Of the seven areas of significant opportunities for information therapy, the one that may offer the greatest potential benefit is that of decision support. In the near future, no major decision for a drug, surgery, or invasive medical test will likely be done without information prescriptions to help the patient participate in the decision. (See page 122 for an example of a decision-support information prescription.)

End-of-Life Care

Information prescriptions to both patients and caregivers as a part of end-of-life care have both huge potential and complex challenges. Emotionally sensitive communication of the right information at the right time can help guide families toward decisions that will best meet their needs through the patient's final days of life.

Checklist for Prescription-Strength Information

☐ Decision-focused. Clearly designed to help consumers arrive at a clinical decision. Explores options and shows evidence bias-free.

☐ Reputable. The sources of the information are from peer-reviewed medical journals and other highly reputable sources.

☐ Reviewed by experts. Lists the medical writer, the medical editor, and the medical reviewer for each topic.

☐ Evidence-based. Where the data exists, information is evidence-based.

☐ Referenced. Clearly references the sources of the information from which the information is derived. These references should also show publication dates.

☐ Up to date. Has dates attached telling when the information was developed and when the last update occurred.

☐ Has a disclosure statement about who funds the information development.

☐ Illustrated. Contains illustrations and other features that help consumers understand.

☐ Emphasizes shared decision making.

☐ Free from commercial bias. Is not trying to sell a specific health or medical product.

☐ Written in easy-to-understand language. Doesn't use heavy medical jargon.

People seldom refuse help, if one offers it in the right way.
A. C. Benson

4

Physician-Prescribed Information Therapy

The purest and most powerful form of information therapy happens when a clinician personally prescribes specific information to help a particular patient better manage a diagnosed problem. Called "physician-prescribed" for convenience, such information prescriptions can be written by any doctor, nurse practitioner, physician assistant, dentist, or other clinician who has a professional relationship with the patient. Information can also come from a coordinated effort by the medical care team.

Clinician-prescribed information, by definition, must be **personalized** to an individual, **targeted** to a "moment in care," and **prescribed** by a health professional who knows the patient.

Personalized

Clinician-prescribed information is presented to a patient by name and with a message that encourages that person to review it. While health information can be found in abundance, information directed to a specific patient is rare. Think about your own response to mail addressed to "Occupant" versus mail addressed to you personally. Marketing researchers have long known that the book you are most likely to open is the one entitled "All about {insert your name here}." Personalization greatly increases the importance that a patient puts on such information and the likelihood that it will be used. In more sophisticated Ix applications, information can be personalized to an individual's interests, readiness for change, reading level, and preferred learning style.

Moments in Care

A "moment in care" is any point in the progression of an illness or medical treatment that calls for a specific decision to be made or a specific behavior to be changed. A moment in care can also denote the transition from primary care to specialty care or at hospital discharge. For each illness, the moments in care can also identify the critical points at which mistakes are most likely to occur.

Much of the success of information therapy is based on the ability to predict when each person approaches a specific moment in care and then provide the information needed to best manage that moment.

❖

Targeted

Clinician-prescribed information can be narrowly targeted to the specific moment in care or medical decision that the patient is facing. Narrow targeting of information both emphasizes the information most important to the patient at that point in care and avoids sending patients into explorations of medical situations that do not apply to them.

Prescribed

Personalized and targeted information has greater impact when it is prescribed by a clinician with whom the patient has an established clinical relationship. That relationship opens a special avenue of communication with the patient. Clinician-prescribed information extends that communication channel beyond the clinic.

Within the parameters of personalized, targeted, and prescribed, clinicians can send information prescriptions to support any or all aspects of the medical care they provide.

This chapter reviews clinician-prescribed Ix opportunities in the context of two dimensions: clinical applications and the degree of technology support.

Clinical applications of information therapy are grouped into three categories:

- **Home care instructions**. Instructions may cover self-care for a minor illness or injury; self-management of chronic illness; guidelines for changing behavior; strengthening exercises and rehab activities; and medication management.

- **Prevention and visit preparation**. In addition to reminders about preventive services, prescriptions can include information about how to prepare for clinic visits, tests, and surgery.

- **Decision-support tools.** These can help consumers make treatment and medical test decisions in an informed way.

Likewise, the technical capabilities of a practice setting are grouped into three categories:

- **Low-tech: All paper.** The clinician either hands out preprinted information in the clinic or uses a checkoff prescription pad to direct the patient to the information on the Internet. No clinic computer is involved or needed.

- **Mid-tech: Paper and wired.** The initial prescription is made on paper and later entered into a computerized system that constructs and sends a message to the patient via e-mail, fax, or mail.

- **High-tech: Wired or wireless.** Clinical information systems assist the clinician in writing the prescription by presenting suggested information links based on clinical information entered into the system for order entry, medical record, billing, or other purposes. Handheld wireless PDAs (personal digital assistants) and other wireless devices can be particularly well-suited for this purpose.

While the ultimate potential of clinician-prescribed information therapy may only be possible through comprehensive EMR (electronic medical record) and order-entry systems, it is encouraging to note that many valuable applications can be delivered with nothing more than a handwritten note on a prescription pad. Regardless of the delivery method, clinician-prescribed information prescriptions can improve both patient satisfaction and the quality of medical care.

Putting Information Therapy Into Practice

What could information therapy in a doctor's practice really look like? Imagine that you are a family practice physician. Your next three patients are described below.

In these cases, information therapy can help you provide your patients with the information they want and need to manage their health problems more effectively. The challenge, of course, is to get the information to them without adding to the already demanding work flow issues of your medical practice. With the help of technology, information therapy is up to the challenge.

Example 1
Mary Morrison

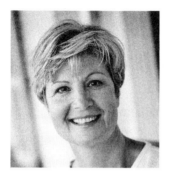

Ix Prescription Pad
(on PDA or EMR)

Chronic Sinusitis
ICD-9 473.9

☐ + Overview

☑ **+ Exams & Tests**

☐ + Tx Overview

☐ + Prevention

☑ **+ Home Treatment**

☑ **+ Medications**

☑ **+ Surgery**

☐ + Other Treatments

☑ **+ Amoxicillin**
   NDC 49884-569
   500-mg tablets, generic

☑ **+ CT Scan for**
   Sinusitis
   CPT 70486, 76375

☑ **+ Ix Search**

Patient: Mary Morrison

History: Mary's sinusitis, which has flared up a few times, is not being controlled with her normal antibiotic, amoxicillin. She has been on the antibiotic for 2 weeks and is getting better slowly. She continues to have facial pain and drainage.

Examination and Tests: Mary's face is tender to the touch over both maxillary sinuses, and the nasal mucosa (tissue) looks swollen and inflamed. No lab tests have been done.

Diagnosis recorded: Chronic Sinusitis (ICD-9 473.9)

Options discussed with Mary:

• Continue on current medication for another 3 weeks.

• Change to new medication: Augmentin and Flonase.

• If there's no improvement after these courses, you explain about additional testing and possible sinus surgery.

You and Mary agree on the following plan:

1. Continue with amoxicillin for an additional 3 weeks. **Rx Prescription recorded: amoxicillin (NDC 49884-569)**

2. Order a CT Scan for 3 weeks from now, which you will cancel if Mary has improved. **Test order recorded: CT Scan (CPT 70486, 76375)**

Information Prescriptions: As you enter Mary's diagnosis and the order for amoxicillin into your PDA or electronic medical record system, the Ix Prescription Pad automatically fills with information prescription options as shown in the box. The checks indicate the Ix prescriptions that you select. You also click on "Ix Search" to send information on Augmentin and Flonase, even though they were not ordered and therefore did not appear automatically.

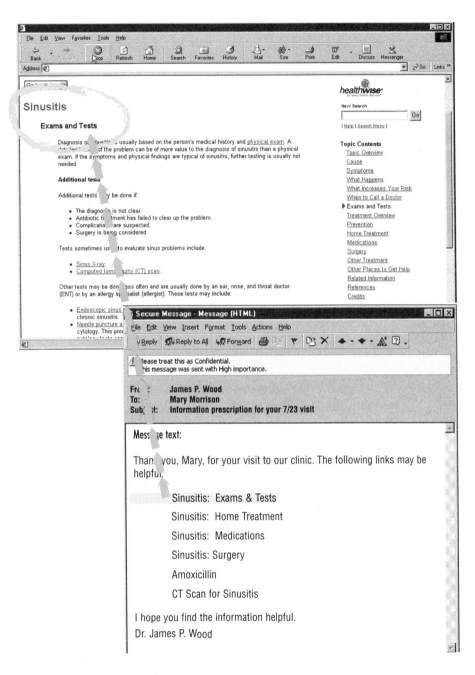

File Edit View Favorites Tools Help

Back   Forward   Stop   Refresh   Home   Search   Favorites   History   Mail   Size   Print   Edit   Discuss   Messenger

Address

healthwise®
for every health decision®

New Search
[   ] Go
| Help | Search Menu |

Sinusitis

Exams and Tests

Diagnosis of sinusitis is usually based on the person's medical history and physical exam. A detailed history of the problem can be of more value to the diagnosis of sinusitis than a physical exam. If the symptoms and physical findings are typical of sinusitis, further testing is usually not needed.

Additional tests

Additional tests may be done if:

- The diagnosis is not clear.
- Antibiotic treatment has failed to clear up the problem.
- Complications are suspected.
- Surgery is being considered.

Tests sometimes used to evaluate sinus problems include:

- Sinus X-ray.
- Computed tomography (CT) scan.

Other tests may be done less often and are usually done by an ear, nose, and throat doctor (ENT) or by an allergy specialist (allergist). These tests may include:

- Endoscopic sinus...
  chronic sinusitis. W...
- Needle puncture a...
  cytology. This proc...

Topic Contents
Topic Overview
Cause
Symptoms
What Happens
What Increases Your Risk
When to Call a Doctor
▶ Exams and Tests
Treatment Overview
Prevention
Home Treatment
Medications
Surgery
Other Treatment
Other Places to Get Help
Related Information
References
Credits

Secure Message - Message (HTML)

File Edit View Insert Format Tools Actions Help

Reply   Reply to All   Forward

⚠ Please treat this as Confidential.
   This message was sent with High importance.

From: **James P. Wood**
To: **Mary Morrison**
Subject: **Information prescription for your 7/23 visit**

Message text:

Thank you, Mary, for your visit to our clinic. The following links may be helpful.

Sinusitis: Exams & Tests

Sinusitis: Home Treatment

Sinusitis: Medications

Sinusitis: Surgery

Amoxicillin

CT Scan for Sinusitis

I hope you find the information helpful.
Dr. James P. Wood

Example 1

To see an example of how this will work, go to
www.informationtherapy.org/examples.

Example 2
Alicia Gomez

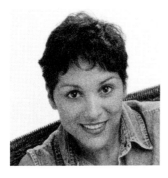

Ix Prescription Pad
(on PDA or EMR)

ACL Injury
ICD-9 844.2

☑ + **Overview**

☑ + **Exams & Tests**

☐ + Tx Overview

☐ + Prevention

☑ + **Home Treatment**

☐ + Medications

☑ + **Surgery Decision**

☐ + Other Treatments

☐ + X-ray: Knee
    CPT 73562

☑ + **Referral Knee**
    (visit prep)

Patient: Alicia Gomez

History: Alicia hurt her knee playing soccer at a picnic yesterday. The swelling is persistent and worsening. Even though the pain is not extreme, Alicia cannot bear weight on the knee. She came into your office on crutches first thing this morning.

Examination and Tests: Your examination finds that Alicia's knee is unstable and that there is a good deal of tenderness and fluid buildup.

You decide to send Alicia for X-rays but to hold off on an MRI for now.

Diagnosis recorded: ACL Injury (ICD-9 844.2)

Options discussed with Alicia:

- Referral to specialist

- Need for X-ray and possible MRI

- Need for surgery versus rehab without surgery

You and Alicia agree on the following plan:

1. Continue the ice, compression, elevation, rest, and crutches.

2. OTC ibuprofen.

3. Order knee X-ray. **Test order recorded: X-ray knee (CPT 73562)**

4. **Referral to sports medicine specialist in 3 days. (Dr. Bill Jones, Provider #55555)**

Information Prescriptions: As checked on Ix Prescription Pad

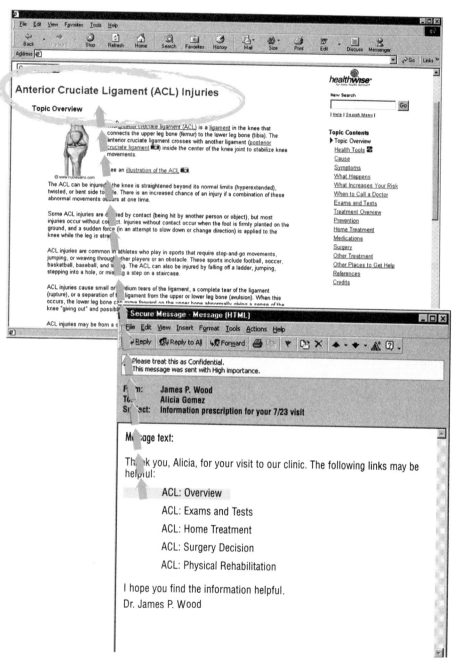

Anterior Cruciate Ligament (ACL) Injuries

Topic Overview

The anterior cruciate ligament (ACL) is a ligament in the knee that connects the upper leg bone (femur) to the lower leg bone (tibia). The anterior cruciate ligament crosses with another ligament (posterior cruciate ligament) inside the center of the knee joint to stabilize knee movements.

© www.nucleusinc.com

See an illustration of the ACL.

The ACL can be injured if the knee is straightened beyond its normal limits (hyperextended), twisted, or bent side to side. There is an increased chance of an injury if a combination of these abnormal movements occurs at one time.

Some ACL injuries are caused by contact (being hit by another person or object), but most injuries occur without contact. Injuries without contact occur when the foot is firmly planted on the ground, and a sudden force (in an attempt to slow down or change direction) is applied to the knee while the leg is straight.

ACL injuries are common in athletes who play in sports that require stop-and-go movements, jumping, or weaving through other players or an obstacle. These sports include football, soccer, basketball, baseball, and skiing. The ACL can also be injured by falling off a ladder, jumping, stepping into a hole, or missing a step on a staircase.

ACL injuries cause small or medium tears of the ligament, a complete tear of the ligament (rupture), or a separation of the ligament from the upper or lower leg bone (avulsion). When this occurs, the lower leg bone can move forward on the upper bone abnormally giving a sense of the knee "giving out" and possibly...

ACL injuries may be from a...

healthwise
for every health decision

New Search

[Go]

| Help | Search Menu |

Topic Contents
▶ Topic Overview
   Health Tools
   Cause
   Symptoms
   What Happens
   What Increases Your Risk
   When to Call a Doctor
   Exams and Tests
   Treatment Overview
   Prevention
   Home Treatment
   Medications
   Surgery
   Other Treatment
   Other Places to Get Help
   References
   Credits

Secure Message - Message [HTML]

File Edit View Insert Format Tools Actions Help

Reply Reply to All Forward

⚑ Please treat this as Confidential.
This message was sent with High importance.

From: James P. Wood
To: Alicia Gomez
Subject: Information prescription for your 7/23 visit

Message text:

Thank you, Alicia, for your visit to our clinic. The following links may be helpful:

ACL: Overview

ACL: Exams and Tests

ACL: Home Treatment

ACL: Surgery Decision

ACL: Physical Rehabilitation

I hope you find the information helpful.
Dr. James P. Wood

Example 2

To see an example of how this will work, go to
www.informationtherapy.org/examples.

Example 3
Jackson Williams

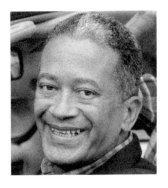

Ix Prescription Pad
(on PDA or EMR)

BPH
ICD-9 600.0

☑ + **Overview**

☐ + Exams & Tests

☐ + Tx Overview

☐ + Prevention

☑ + **Home Treatment**

☑ + **Medications**

☑ + **Surgery Decision**

☐ + Other Treatments

☑ + **PSA Test** CPT 84152

☑ + **Hytrin**
(terazosin)
NDC 0074-3806-13
2-mg capsules, 100

Patient: Jackson Williams

History: Jackson's long history of urinary problems has gradually worsened. The strength of his stream has decreased significantly. He is waking up to urinate two to three times a night and often has a problem starting urination when he first gets up in the morning. Because of some dribbling, he occasionally gets some irritation under his foreskin. He is bothered by all of these symptoms, and he's also worried that the symptoms may mean he has prostate cancer.

Examination and Tests:

* The AUA Symptom Index score of 15: mid- to high-moderate

* Blood drawn to repeat a prostate-specific antigen (PSA). **Test order recorded: PSA Test (CPT 84152)**

* A digital rectal exam: enlarged but without any abnormalities

Diagnosis recorded: BPH, Benign Prostatic Hyperplasia (ICD-9 600.0)

Options discussed with Jackson:

* Agree on plan if inability to urinate occurs or if pain develops.

* Start alpha-blocker medication.

* Surgery (TURP or TUIP) to remove obstruction of the urethra.

You and Jackson agree on the following plan:

1. Emphasize home treatment.

2. Prescribe terazosin (Hytrin) for 4-week trial. **Rx Prescription recorded: Hytrin (NDC 0074-3806-13)**

3. Review the information about surgery, drugs, or watchful waiting.

Information Prescriptions: As checked on Ix Prescription Pad

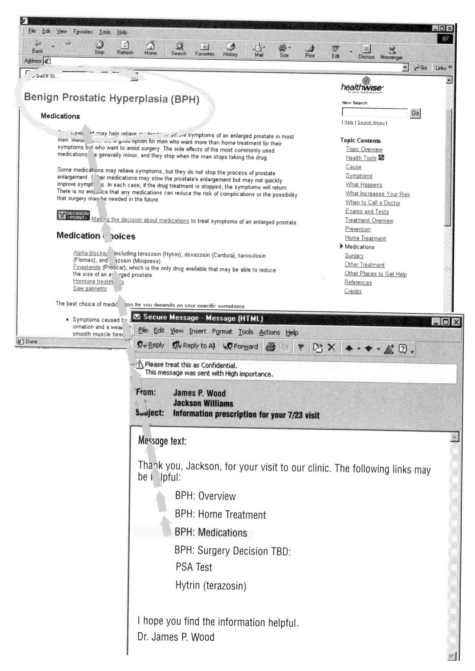

Example 3

To see an example of how this will work, go to
www.informationtherapy.org/examples.

Educating Patients: The Physician's Perspective

The idea of physicians giving information to help their patients better manage disease is as old as medicine. Every physician does it in every clinical visit. Until now, however, the exchange of information between physicians and patients has been plagued by several major limitations.

Limitations

- **Too little time to keep up to date**. One of the greatest challenges for physicians is keeping up to date on clinical knowledge. So much new information comes out each week on medical treatments, diagnostic tests, medications, and surgical techniques that physicians have to devote nearly all of their training time to staying clinically up to date. They don't have much time to study new ways to educate patients.

  The strategy physicians most often use is to tell the patient what the physician thinks is most important to remember and do. It sounds simple enough. Physicians are likely to do this orally, without a checklist, and with no way of knowing how much the patient understands. Because the information is spoken only, there is no easy way to judge its completeness or its consistency across patients with similar conditions. This type of patient education also does not allow for the information and patient knowledge to build from visit to visit.

- **Too little time to educate patients**. The pressure of waiting room backlogs and mountains of paperwork often pushes physicians to rush the patient education portion of the visit. There may be time only for a quick presentation of the most important things to remember and no time to check with the patient on how much was understood.

- **Overreliance on patient memory**. Physicians rarely provide patients the means to record the information that is orally presented. Patients are given complex directions in a medical language they often don't understand at a time when they are likely to be anxious and unwell. It is a wonder that patients remember any of the information conveyed once they get home.

- **Patient indifference to information**. There will always be patients who have little or no interest in understanding their conditions or participating in their care. In these cases, efforts at patient education may seem like a waste of time. Fortunately, most patients today are ready to learn about their options and help with their care.

- **"Nonwired" patients**. Even without e-mail or Web access, however, nonwired patients can still get information prescriptions. Options include access by a friend or relative (signed released may be required); access on a "patient station" in a waiting room, using a computer and printer; a printed version handed out in the clinic; information printed and mailed to the patient; and information electronically sent to a call center where the patient can call for the information. Nonwired patients can also find information at their local libraries with the help of medical or reference librarians.

Information therapy can help physicians overcome these limitations. It can also make their efforts at patient education more efficient in their medical practice and more valuable to their patients.

Incentives

Doctors are smart people. Few physicians will change their practice routines without a good set of compelling reasons. A physician must clearly see how a change will result in better medicine for the patient. If that cause-and-effect relationship is not clear, the change has little chance of happening. While most physicians support the basic idea that a better-informed patient results in better care, there is little evidence that physicians are willing

---

Clinician Hopes for Information Therapy

- *Help meet my patient's expectations*

- *Help my patient understand*

- *Help my patient follow instructions*

- *Help my patient be involved in decisions when appropriate*

- *Help me practice better care*

- *Help me stay on schedule*

---

to significantly increase either office visit time or patient education budgets to achieve greater patient understanding. For physicians to support a change in practice toward information therapy, that change must result in more than just a better-informed patient.

- **Information therapy must save time**. Physicians value what helps them stick to their schedules. "Getting behind" is a considerable stressor that physicians face every day. The classic dilemma is whether to spend more time helping a patient understand the treatment options while knowing that with every minute spent in education, the waiting room backlog increases. Presenting patients with efficiently constructed information prescriptions that are directly relevant to their conditions and treatment plans would result in better medicine while helping the physician avoid waiting room problems and "getting-behind" stress.

- **Information therapy must build loyalty**. Physicians increasingly recognize that many of their patients are asking for more information than a physician can provide during a scheduled appointment. For many patients, the ability of a doctor to meet their information needs has become as important a loyalty factor as the doctor's medical expertise and bedside manner. By providing personalized information prescriptions, the clinician can guarantee a more positive approval rating and increased patient loyalty. Greater patient approval ratings translate directly to bonus pay for physicians in some physician groups.[1]

- **Information therapy must solve the Internet conundrum**. Physicians are often stymied by their "Internet" patients—those who refer to reams of Internet downloads from unknown Web sites and then ask their doctor for an opinion about the information. There is simply no reasonable way to respond to these requests within the time available. Information prescriptions change the dynamics entirely. By prescribing information known to be of high quality, the physician returns to a prominent place in the information/education loop with the patient. If patients get the information they want and need from their doctors, they may not bring stacks of Internet printouts to their next visit.

To gain these benefits, physicians will need to steel their resolve: the introduction of information therapy to a practice will not come pain-free. Investments of time and dollars are needed up front to make information therapy possible. However, for most physicians, the potential of increased quality, saved time, patient loyalty, and regained control are sufficient to justify the move toward information therapy—as long as it can be seamlessly added to the work flow of the practice.

In the future, there may be another potential incentive for physicians to support information prescriptions: they may get paid for it. Until now, physicians have rarely stopped to ask why their patient education services have gone unrecognized in reimbursement formulas. However, once the subject is raised, it is not hard to gain support for the idea that information prescriptions should be valued economically as well as clinically. The potential for reimbursing for information prescriptions is extensively reviewed in Chapter 8.

Act Now: Get Started With Information Prescriptions

Any clinician can begin making information prescriptions with a few hours' time investment and virtually no financial investment. (Internet access is required.) Here's how:

1. Create a priority list. List the top 10 to 15 medical topics your patients want or need information on during a typical week's practice.

2. Review what's out there. Go to several public access Web sites that you trust to have good information about each topic, and review the information that each has on your priority topics.

3. Choose your source. For each topic, write down the URL (Uniform Resource Locator, the unique Web page address) that gets right to the information you want your patients to see.

4. Share the information. When you see a patient who needs that information, supplement your verbal explanation by including the appropriate URL on your prescription pad and suggesting that the patient review it within the next few days.

Information therapy can be as easy as that. If you pick the targeted topics well, find good sites to recommend, and are diligent in using them, handwritten information prescriptions can make a big difference to your practice. Granted, the handwritten prescription approach takes a highly motivated clini-

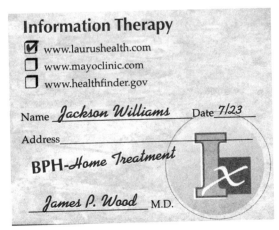

Information Therapy

☑ www.laurushealth.com
☐ www.mayoclinic.com
☐ www.healthfinder.gov

Name _Jackson Williams_ Date _7/23_

Address_____

BPH-Home Treatment

James P. Wood M.D.

cian. It takes a little time to write the prescription, more time to document it in the record (optional), and still more time to periodically check to see if the referenced URLs are still active and still appropriate for your patients. While many physicians are already using this approach, many more are waiting for a better technological solution.

We want to make a prediction: The number and value of information prescriptions will multiply rapidly the moment that computerized order entry becomes mainstream. With either wireless clinician PDAs (personal digital assistants), tablet PCs, or exam room desktop access for medication prescriptions, lab test orders, and medical record entry, the process of adding a clinically relevant information order will become almost automatic.

Consider the case of Mary Morrison's sinusitis. Using his PDA, Dr. Wood would have already accomplished the following:

- Tapped on Mary's name and ID number to identify the patient

- Tapped on the name, dose, and duration of the prescribed medication

- Tapped on Chronic Sinusitis for visit billing purposes (with the appropriate ICD-9 code attached to it)

- Tapped to order the Sinusitis CT Scan

- Tapped to indicate that a revisit is to be scheduled

Next, Dr. Wood taps on the information therapy icon. At that point the PDA displays all of the following for selection, confirmation, or change:

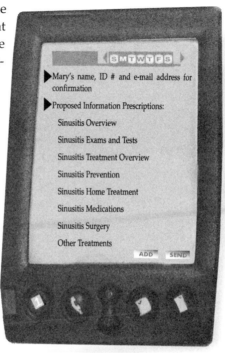

- Mary's name, ID number, and e-mail address for confirmation

- Proposed Information Prescriptions:

  - Sinusitis Overview

  - Sinusitis Exams and Tests

  - Sinusitis Treatment Overview

  - Sinusitis Prevention

  - Sinusitis Home Treatment

  - Sinusitis Medications

  - Sinusitis Surgery

  - Other Treatments

  - Amoxicillin

  - CT Scan for Sinusitis

- Send visit prep package prior to revisit.

Dr. Wood taps to select the "Home Treatment," "Sinusitis Surgery," and "CT Scan" prescriptions. Finally, he taps to okay the information prescription links.

With just a few taps beyond his normal work flow, Dr. Wood has sent a personalized, targeted, and prescribed information prescription on its way. Not only that, but the information prescription is automatically documented and attached to Mary's electronic medical record. Finally, without any additional effort by Dr. Wood or his staff, the system is already poised to send Mary a second information prescription 3 days before her planned revisit in 3 weeks.

With less than a minute of review and prescription "writing," Dr. Wood has saved Mary the anxiety, time, and effort she would have had to spend hunting for similar information on the Internet; he has also saved himself the time reviewing her downloads and battling the misinformation she might have found in her search. Mary is better informed, better prepared, and more likely to be satisfied with her encounter.

Home Care Prescriptions

A practice might choose to implement an Ix application for home care instructions as a quick and easy way to get started with information prescriptions. The application could focus on as few or as many of the common needs for home treatment information as desired. Depending on the practice specialty, physicians and nurses would preselect specific self-care and self-management information prescriptions for inclusion in the system. The set of home care instructions could include any or all of the following:

- Recovery following injury (rest, ice, elevation, etc.)

- Restrengthening following injury (stretching, exercise, etc.)

- Nutrition, fitness, and stress management activities

- Specific disease management tasks (glucose monitoring, etc.)

- Medication management instructions

All such prescriptions can be developed in advance, periodically reviewed, and ordered from a list either by the clinician on a PDA or by the office staff from the clinician's notes. These prescriptions can be waiting for the patient by the time he or she gets home from the clinic. Since home-care instructions are often only a few pages, in-office printing for patients without Internet access or e-mail is also possible.

Preventive Services Prescriptions

Medical practices that use computer applications for visit scheduling, preventive services monitoring, test scheduling, or procedure scheduling may wish to use that information to trigger preventive services prescriptions.

- Immunization reminders can be triggered by combining age and immunization records. The reminder can carry with it any of the following functions:

  - Notice that the immunization appears due

  - Information about the risks and benefits of the immunization

  - Cost information and acceptable methods of payment

  - Hours that the office is open for immunization

  - Other locations where immunizations are available

  - Link to automated scheduling system (if one exists)

- Allergy alerts can include seasonal notices predicting pollen blooms, pollution alerts, or other environmental changes that might trigger increased preventive strategies for "at-risk" individuals.

- Preventive services reminders for mammograms, cholesterol tests, eye exams, and other recommended screenings can be customized to match the needs of each patient and staggered to match the scheduling availability of the clinic. (Using Internet messaging, these reminders can be better targeted, more effective, and less expensive than the practice of sending birthday card reminders for needed preventive services.)

- Encouraging words can include notices to remind patients to renew efforts toward fitness or dietary plans that may be noted in their records.

Visit Prep Prescriptions

Information about the reason for a visit, collected by the scheduling clerk at the time a visit is scheduled, can be used to send a visit preparation message to the patient. Visit prep messages can include any or all of the following, which may result in a more productive clinic visit:

- Reminder of the time and location for visit (link to map/directions) and request to call if there is a need to reschedule or cancel

- Symptom review and information-gathering questionnaire related to the reason for the visit (for doctor-patient review in the visit)

- Home treatment suggestions related to the reason for visit

- Patient history form (new or update)

Decision-Support Prescriptions

The term "decision support" simply refers to information that helps a patient decide among treatment or test options. The most valuable information a clinician can prescribe is information that helps a patient reach a better treatment decision. Shared medical decision making in which the patient learns the costs, risks, and benefits of the treatment options and the clinician learns the related values and preferences of the patient inevitably leads to better medical decisions.

Without information prescriptions, shared medical decision making is difficult to support in most practice settings. There is simply not enough time to fully inform patients in time for them to participate effectively in decisions. While the concept of shared decision making is well accepted by the medical profession, a study looking at the patient's role in clinical decision making found that only 9 percent of medical decisions could be rated as completely informed decisions.[2]

With a decision-support Ix application in place, however, shared decision making can become the standard operating procedure. Any medical practice can begin by prescribing decision-support information for just a few treatment decisions that are important to patients and come up frequently. Clinics supported by wireless PDA systems or other automation can offer decision support for decisions about referrals, medical tests, medications, and surgery and other treatments.

The challenge for each decision-support opportunity is to get the information to patients "at the right time" to help with their decision. When there is a scheduled revisit at which major clinical decisions will be made, sending the information before the second visit works fine. However, scheduling revisits for most routine decisions is clearly not practical. The inevitable result is that the decision is made either by the clinician without the patient's informed participation or by the patient based on information reviewed after the visit but without the benefit of the clinician's help at the time of the decision.

Some physicians build a level of patient choice into their practice by sending the patient home with the information needed to make a final decision. Patients review the information, think about their preferences, and then call the clinic to ask that the medication be prescribed or the procedure be scheduled. While this solution gets close to shared decision making, a far better solution is to get the information to the patient in advance of the visit. "Information triggers" that can predict what decisions patients might be facing in their next visit are discussed at length in the next chapter on system-prescribed information.

Preadmission Prescriptions

Hospitalization is a major life event for a patient. One information therapy need for each patient scheduled for hospital admission is a customized and personalized "survivor's guide" to the hospital. Yes, there are many generic "hospital survivor guides" in print, but most patients enter the hospital without seeing one. If the admitting physician could prescribe such a guide, specifically customized for the individual patient, presumably much of the anxiety and concern surrounding hospital stays could be avoided and many of the factors leading to improved outcomes and higher patient satisfaction could be set in place.

Such a survivor's guide would combine three sets of information important to the patient:

1. **Diagnosis and treatment**. Information about the specific diagnosis and treatment (much like that in the decision-support prescriptions discussed above but extending to each specific test or procedure included in the treatment plan).

2. **Hospital guidelines**. Information about making the hospital stay more comfortable, including what the patient can bring, who can visit and when, and what the patient's rights are.

3. **The patient's role in recovery**. Information about what the patient can do to help make the treatment successful and to minimize the risk of medical errors.

Ix Assessments: Is Your Clinic Ready?

How can you tell if your clinic is ready to implement information therapy? Try completing an Ix assessment. Whether an independent consultant, the clinic's administrative staff, or the physicians themselves conduct the assessment, it can lay out a course of action that will lead to the full integration of information therapy within the practice. A well-done assessment can identify both opportunities for success and barriers to overcome.

Please note:

Outlines for each of the four components in the Ix Clinic Assessment can be found in Appendix B beginning on page 221.

Look first for "low-hanging fruit." Starting with easy implementations that quickly yield high-value returns will build momentum and the commitment to support more in-depth implementations later. A good assessment will help a clinic focus its start-up Ix initiatives in areas that bring the most value to the practice and its patients with the least risk of failure.

Your goal: Identify the applications and issues that will make or break information therapy (the "killer apps" and "application killers").

"Killer apps" are Ix applications so valuable that once they are in place, you will not be able to take them away from the practice without sacrificing quality of care and efficiency. For example, an Ix service that significantly increases the percentage of heart attack survivors who make the transition from hospital to home on the correct medication plan might be considered a "killer app."

"Application killers" are the obstacles that can prevent a killer app from full implementation. It is just as important to identify the potential barriers as the potential benefits when building the implementation plan. Such barriers can be political, legal, economic, or even emotional. For example, if an Ix application creates embarrassment for a doctor (even once), its chances for large-scale implementation are significantly reduced.

A full Ix assessment entails four components:

1. Clinic Overview

2. Physician, Nurse, and Staff Interviews

3. Technical Assessment

4. Patient Survey

An analysis of the findings in each of the four assessment components should lead to a report of conclusions that looks at implementing an Ix plan from three different perspectives:

1. **Quality:** Which information prescriptions will best help the patients and improve quality?

2. **Work flow:** Which approaches will most help practice efficiency and work flow?

3. **Technology:** Which applications fit best with the information technology in place or planned for clinic implementation?

Ix Opportunities From the Quality Perspective

Chapter 3 identified and outlined the seven opportunities for information therapy: self-care, prevention, self-triage, visit preparation, shared decision making, chronic illness self-management, and end-of-life care. The priorities for development in each of these areas differ for every medical practice based on the specialty, patient mix, and skill set of the staff.

The assessment will help you focus on the needs of the patient for information therapy. Consider a surgical practice. A surgical practice usually entails few "walk-ins," fairly good previsit information from referring physicians, a clear diagnosis, and at least a tentative set of potential treatment options. In such a setting, patients have less need for information about self-care, prevention, and self-triage but more need for information about visit or procedure preparation and shared decision making.

Sending information prescriptions prior to a visit will help patients ask better questions, give better answers to the physician's questions, and be better prepared to consider the surgery decision. In addition to better preparation for surgery, the positive outcomes may include greater understanding and acceptance of risks, which will result in improved satisfaction and potentially lower risk for malpractice claims.

Likewise, for a specialty like endocrinology, it may be possible to identify a dozen information prescriptions for self-management of chronic disease that meet the information needs of a large percentage of a physician's practice. By focusing on the educational issues to which the physician already devotes the most time, information prescriptions can greatly improve the effectiveness and value of the education without extending visit time or cost.

Formalizing invitations to participate in self-management classes or Web-based interactive programs through information prescriptions can greatly increase the number of patients who benefit from such programs. Improvements in quality of care and treatment outcomes should follow.

Even a family medicine practice that sees patients of all ages and socioeconomic situations with a broad range of problems can identify conditions that arise again and again each week or season. Focusing on those conditions, plus helping patients with self-care, self-triage, and visit preparation, can provide the biggest value contribution by helping to save time and meeting patients' needs. In many such cases, a degree of automation can be remarkably helpful. Allowing the clinician to choose from a broad-ranging set of information prescriptions prepared in advance by experts in each medical specialty expands the impact of information therapy and helps patients find better care and healthier outcomes.

Ix Opportunities From the Work Flow Perspective

Assessing work flow—how the work gets done—is critical to introducing information therapy into practice. If information therapy increases the time spent per patient or reduces the number of patients helped per day, it won't survive.

Work flow can make or break a clinic. Anything that disrupts work flow, no matter how beneficial to the patient, exacts a steep price by reducing the number of patients that can be seen in a day or by requiring additional resources. A work flow assessment looks at how many people must interact with each patient and how many discrete tasks each individual must perform to achieve a successful visit.

Information therapy applications that increase the number of steps or staff required to achieve a successful patient visit are not likely to succeed. However, in many cases, Ix applications combined with work flow redesign or clinic automation can actually streamline operations and result in increased clinic productivity, greater patient satisfaction, and better medical outcomes. The assessment should examine the practice to uncover potential opportunities for Ix innovations in those areas.

Ix Opportunities From the Technology Perspective

The assessment also looks at how the technology infrastructure within a clinic can support Ix prescriptions. Once a medical practice prepares to move to computerized medication prescriptions, physician order entry, or electronic medical records, the additional effort it takes to add an Ix service is quite small. (The time to convert to computer-aided systems may be upon you for other reasons: recent proposals by the Institute of Medicine suggest that handwritten prescriptions and other orders should be largely abandoned by 2010.)[3] With further advances to a wireless handheld chart, writing information prescriptions will become virtually effortless for practicing physicians.

Innovator Profiles

The remainder of this chapter presents three profiles of people and organizations that are currently delivering clinician-prescribed information therapy. While in many ways these innovator profiles focus on pioneers, they also represent what we think will soon become commonplace and mainstream in American health care. The profiles include:

A physician. Steven L. Schneider, MD, is a family practice physician who has implemented the philosophy of information therapy into his practice with no technological assistance.

A virtual clinic. Doctor Goodwell connects physicians and their patients via videoconferencing at the workplace. This virtual clinic has placed a strong emphasis on information prescriptions and informed decision making.

A decision-support service. Health Dialog allows nurse care counselors to help empower and inform patients to make better health decisions and avoid medical errors.

For each innovator highlighted in these pages, there are many others now developing, implementing, and evaluating Ix applications.

Steven L. Schneider, MD

Dr. Schneider is a family practice physician in Boise, Idaho. He founded the Idaho Wellness Center in 1980, an innovative family practice based on prevention, self-care, and self-responsibility. The Center is now a part of Primary Health, a 60-physician group practice. Dr. Schneider is also chief medical officer for Healthwise, Incorporated.

Dr. Schneider has been prescribing Web-based information to his patients since 1996 when the Healthwise Communities Project launched a consumer health Web site for the community. He uses a prescription pad to write out the Web address and topic he'd like his patient to review.

Q & A with Dr. Schneider

Q: *What percent of your patients get information prescriptions? How much time does it take?*

A: About 30 percent get them and it takes about 2 minutes to write and explain the prescription.

Q: *How many patients actually look up the information?*

A: About 70 percent of patients follow through. I try to match the information to the patient's interests.

Q: *How do you work with patients who have no Internet access?*

A: We have a computer in the waiting room that patients can use.

Q: *What's next for information therapy at Primary Health?*

A: We want to integrate information therapy into an electronic medical record. We have an initiative to standardize and improve quality of care among the various doctors. We'll use information therapy as the patient component of that standardization.

Q: *What makes you invest your time in information therapy?*

A: There is no doubt that this helps me practice better medicine. I had a long-time patient who was recently diagnosed with diabetes. I gave him an information prescription to look up the diabetes topic on the community Web site. He came in 4 weeks later for follow-up care, and when I walked into the room, he already had his shoes and socks off. He told me he read in the topic that I was going to have to check his feet, so he prepared for it. When it's busy at my practice, it's easy to miss important steps. So, it was good to have that patient work with me to get the best care.

Doctor Goodwell
www.doctorgoodwell.net

Doctor Goodwell is an Internet-based virtual clinic service that connects doctors with their patients outside of the traditional clinic setting. Doctor Goodwell is a development of Overlake Hospital Medical Center in Bellevue, Washington. The project has been developed in close collaboration with Microsoft and is currently used by a subset of Microsoft employees in the Bellevue area.

The company's "virtual visits" allow for two-way, video-enabled office visits so that employees at work can consult with doctors to discuss, diagnose, and treat minor medical issues. Doctors can deliver information prescriptions to online patients. Patients can also use secure messaging to consult with doctors regarding health concerns and to schedule virtual appointments. The service is designed to eliminate the need for visits when a quick question and answer or medication refill request is all that is required.

Company founders believe that the fundamental benefit of Doctor Goodwell is the improved productivity gained by eliminating the loss of 2 to 3 hours of employee time typically needed for simple office visits. There are also significant quality improvements built into the system, such as the information prescriptions that can be simultaneously transmitted during the virtual visit. In addition, the clinics gain clinical visit revenue without extra staffing and related facility costs.

Ix Applications

As part of the automated process that employees use to schedule virtual visits with their doctors, they must identify the main reason for the visit. The system uses that reason for visit to select content from a central knowledge base that is sent to the patient with confirmation of the scheduled virtual visit.

In addition, the secure messaging system includes a function that makes it easy for physicians to attach links to medical content to their responses to the patient. The links are automatically suggested by the system based on the nature of the patient's request. The physician reviews all information links before the message is delivered. In implementation of the virtual clinic system, about 65 percent of the visits resulted in information prescriptions of relevant content.

Health Dialog
www.healthdialog.com

Health Dialog, of Boston, is a condition management company focused on improving the quality and reducing the cost of health care through more informed patient-physician dialogues.

Health Dialog was founded in 1997 in close cooperation with the Foundation for Informed Medical Decision Making. Founded 8 years earlier by physicians John E. Wennberg (Director, Center for Evaluative Clinical Sciences at Dartmouth Medical School) and Albert G. Mulley Jr. (Division Chief, General Medicine at Massachusetts General Hospital), the Foundation develops evidence-based coaching materials and promotes the use of Shared Decision-Making® in medicine. Health Dialog is the exclusive commercial distributor of all products and medical content created by the Foundation.

Working through health plans and employers, Health Dialog first identifies individuals with chronic conditions or those facing major medical decisions, and then provides them the information and coaching they need to have well-informed discussions with their clinicians.

The Health Dialog service includes a 24/7 telephone-based network staffed with experienced nurses, dieticians, and respiratory therapists who act as "health coaches" for consumers. The health coaches rely on an advanced information system platform that includes proprietary information developed by the Foundation. The coaching network is supplemented by Web services that allow the consumer to access and review the same information available to the health coaches.

Health Dialog's core strategy is based on evidence that suggests that Shared Decision-Making® in medical care leads to both improved outcomes and lower costs. Health Dialog's products and services help individuals work with their clinicians to make the best care decisions. By providing the latest clinical evidence in the context of decision support that encourages patient preference, Health Dialog is able to facilitate decisions that result in high consumer satisfaction.

Ix Applications

Health Dialog's health coaches provide information to consumers from the same database they use when talking to consumers about their conditions. They can print and mail the information or provide Web links. Particular focus is placed on prescribing Health Dialog's Shared Decision-Making® videotapes, Web modules, and printed decision tools to people who need them. The health coaches then use their coaching skills to provide consumers with the confidence needed to make the most appropriate care decisions.

Questions From Clinicians

Q: *As a primary care physician, I see patients come to me every day with stacks of information gathered from the Internet. Some of the information is helpful, but a lot of it is not. I have only seconds to evaluate which is which for each patient. It is an impossible situation. How will information therapy help?*

A: Information won't work as therapy unless you trust that the information is high-quality, accurate, and targeted to match the needs of your patient. With Ix prescriptions, you both control the source of the information and select the information that matches the patient's needs. Even when you have not fully reviewed the information, limit it to what has been reviewed by medical experts that you trust. To meet prescription-strength standards, information must be up to date, referenced to the source literature, and reviewed by well-credentialed medical experts. If that structure for a single source exists, it can actually save you time as well as provide a tool that allows you to educate your patients better than you would otherwise have time to do.

Q: *My time per visit is already too short. How will I find more time to do information therapy?*

A: Information therapy can *save* you time. Proper explanations of medical conditions or treatment plans can often take more time than you have to give. Even when you do take the time, patients often remember very little of the explanations once they get home. Writing an information prescription can add only seconds to the clinic visit work flow and leaves a lasting record for the patient to return to at any time. By using the clinic time you *do* have to motivate the patient to read the information and to follow the self-management guidelines or decision-support steps included, you can better inform the patient and get home in time for dinner.

Q: *What about my patients who don't have e-mail?*

A: With secure messaging systems, patients without permanent e-mail addresses can still benefit from information therapy. A patient can access the information from any Internet connection. Many public libraries provide free access. For greater convenience, clinics can install Internet access in the waiting room and restrict use to Ix purposes. Information can also be printed and handed to the patient, although at a substantially higher investment in time and cost. Information prescriptions can also be "filled" via a toll-free nurse advice line, providing you have access to it too.

Q: *What about my patients who don't read or who don't speak or read English?*

A: People who don't read or don't speak English often have access to kin or support networks who will help them understand needed information. You may ask your nonreading patients if they want the information to go to a support person. Another mechanism is to connect patients with a toll-free nurse advice line.

Q: *Many of my patients have co-morbidities. I could send them too much information. How do I decide what to send first?*

A: Co-morbidities complicate the patient's information needs. Over time, information prescriptions will become sophisticated enough to target information for combinations of conditions. Until then, it is best to let the patient judge how much to include in an information prescription.

Q: *What are the privacy and security risks of physician-prescribed information services?*

A: An information prescription written by a clinician to a specific patient requires the same level of privacy protection and security as any other personal medical information under the HIPAA (Health Insurance Portability and Accountability Act) regulations. E-mail systems may not be secure enough. A secure messaging system provides adequate privacy protection and security.

Q: *How do I know whether a patient is "ready" for an Ix prescription?*

A: Some patients may not want an information prescription. If in doubt, just ask. As in any other part of medical care, the patient can decline a recommended treatment. However, if you recommend the information, most patients will be glad to have it.

Q: *Are legal notices needed on each information prescription?*

A: There is little or no case law on the subject. However, to be safe, each information prescription should include a legal notice to inform the recipient of its limitations. Because state laws differ, a local attorney should review and modify the statement as needed. The following statement is just one example:

> *Please note: While the information presented above is often helpful for people with your interests, it may not be appropriate for your specific condition. The information is provided for educational purposes only and not intended to be a substitute for professional medical advice.*

Questions From Consumers

Q: *Does information therapy limit what I can look up on the Internet?*

A: Not at all. An Ix prescription lets your physician or health center direct you to information that is high-quality, well-referenced, and related to your condition and "moment in care." It does not limit you from going to other sources in search of additional information. However, keep in mind that your physician may have little time to review information from other Internet sources.

Q: *How do I know I can trust the information received in an information prescription?*

A: Most people will trust information if it is recommended by their physician. The physician's recommendation is extremely important in establishing the credibility of the information. In addition, prescribed information should be well-documented as to source, authors, reviewers, and date of last update.

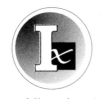

Form follows function.
Louis Henri Sullivan

5

System-Prescribed Information Therapy

Imagine how it would feel to people if the health care system seemed to be working for them rather than against them. Envision a system that did far more for patients than merely send bills or complicated instructions on how to use complicated benefits or tell patients who they can or cannot see. With information therapy, it is possible for a system to truly support its members in obtaining better health care.

> System-prescribed information therapy uses "standing orders" for information. Prescription-Strength Information is automatically delivered to a person in or entering a specific "moment in care."

Standing orders in medicine are a physician's order that can be exercised by other health care workers when predetermined conditions have been met. They "usually name the condition and prescribe the action to be taken in caring for the patient."[1] System-prescribed information therapy (Ix) is similar to standing orders for medications or medical tests in that information is automatically prescribed based on specific information about a particular patient or person. These standing information orders include both the content links and the message that conveys the links to the patient. By consistently connecting Prescription-Strength Information to specific moments in care, system-prescribed information therapy will have a dramatic impact on the value, cost, and quality of health care.

The Case for Standing Information Orders

There is a certain beauty to the idea of creating and employing standing information orders, but there are challenges too. The timeliness and consistency of standing orders are the central benefits of system-prescribed information therapy. The biggest challenge lies in accurately predicting the individual's specific moment in care.

Timeliness and Consistency

Information prescriptions have the most value when they are delivered at the right time. That usually means in time to influence a medical decision. In the average clinic visit, the time that elapses between the patient's presentation of symptoms and the physician's prescription of treatment is under 15 minutes. In many cases, the patient will need more time than that to fully understand the options, consider his or her preferences, and contribute to the clinical decision. For many of the most important moments in care, the time allowed in an office visit simply does not support shared decision making. In order for the patient to fully participate in decision making, needed information should reach the patient in advance of the decision-making visit.

Faced with time constraints within the clinic visit and with a general lack of needed information coming from the clinician to the patient, many tech-savvy consumers will go online in search of information in advance of each doctor visit. It's a hunt fraught with peril.

In Chapter 2, we highlighted some of the misinformation that is available on the Internet (see pages 19 to 21). We also reported the three main problems that RAND Health found in its assessment of health-related information on the Internet:[2]

1. **Search engines can let you down**. Internet search engines are "only moderately efficient in locating information on a particular health topic. More than half of consumers who use the Internet report that they spend about a half hour looking for health information. . . ." And, what you end up with depends upon where you begin. "(Search engines') variability in performance suggests that the likelihood of finding the information one needs, on the topic of one's choice, will depend on where one starts."

2. **There are significant gaps in the availability of key information**. Expert panels found that only half of the topics important for consumers were covered more than minimally:

> Consumers using the Internet may have a difficult time finding complete and accurate information on a health problem. If people are relying on the Internet to make treatment decisions, including whether to seek care, deficiencies in information could negatively influence consumer decisions.

3. **What's that you say?** Most Web-based health information is difficult for the average consumer to understand: "The reading level of most Web-based material is quite high."

Let us add a further assumption to these findings: Even well-informed patients are likely to experience a communications breakdown with their physicians when presenting information gleaned from the Internet. Many physicians dislike patient-proffered Internet downloads. The physician must question where the patient is getting the information. If the physician does not trust the source or know the content, he or she is not likely to support it. And, certainly, there is too little time for the physician to review it and respond during the visit. For many providers, health information from the Web further complicates an already complex interaction.

The remedy to these hazards lies in the physician and the health care system taking a proactive stance. The solution is to send information that the physician knows and trusts to the patient in advance of the visit, using "standing information orders." Vetted and suitable information can then become a shared foundation for the doctor-patient discussion about treatment options and next steps.

The logic of system-prescribed information/standing information orders is straightforward:

- Each moment in care is defined within a hierarchy of clinical situations with common characteristics and information needs.

- Clinical qualifiers are used to add content that applies only in specific clinical situations.

- **Information triggers** are used to predict when a person is in or approaching a moment in care. Each information trigger is associated with specific links to information that are useful in managing the moment in care.

- Information about the patient is used to send a **tailored message**.

- **Blocking factors** are used to prevent inappropriate messages from going out.

- The information is delivered in a **prescription** sent to the patient by e-mail and secure messaging systems.

Standing information orders can be prescribed for every scheduled appointment (based on the "reason for the visit"), every lab test, X-ray, or other diagnostic procedure (based on the CPT code and result), and every preventive services visit or chronic disease checkup that has not occurred on schedule. In these situations, information can be delivered automatically regardless of whether or not the physician remembers to do it, whether or not the clinic is an hour behind schedule, and whether or not the patient thinks to ask for it.

Currently, even though health care consumerism is growing and a majority of Americans are Web-connected and looking for health information on the Internet, fewer than one in ten clinical decisions made by doctor and patient are made with the patient fully informed.[3] Through standing orders that send information in advance of visits or clinical decision points, the rate of informed decision making should climb. The combined strengths of timeliness and consistency make system-prescribed information therapy a powerful force.

Accuracy

Here's the rub. The single greatest challenge of system-prescribed information therapy comes in the difficulty of accurately predicting an individual's specific moment in care. While no single set of codes or structured language is focused on moments in care, reliable and accurate medical coding can help. Unfortunately, getting to accurate coding is not as easy as it might seem. (The issue of inaccurate coding is further discussed in the "Information Triggers" section that begins on page 83.)

Because of a lack of confidence in the accuracy of predicting moments in care, system-produced information prescriptions must be broader and less precise than those prescribed by the patient's own clinician. To avoid legal concerns with medical practice regulations, the messages that are not based on standing orders from the patient's own clinician must be written in a less prescriptive manner. These concerns, along with the issues of privacy protection and confidentiality, are discussed on page 215.

Moments in Care

A moment in care is any specific, identifiable point in the diagnosis or treatment of a condition. Particularly important moments in care occur at transition points, such as a transfer of care from a family physician to a specialist or at hospital discharge. However, many smaller moments in care occur with every medical decision that the patient and physician must ponder and act on. Large or small, each moment in care can be associated with key decisions, potential errors in care, and patient behaviors that can improve or threaten medical outcomes.

While every moment in care for every patient is unique, in practice, moments in care must be grouped into categories. "Moment-in-care" thinking can help Ix planners develop targeted information prescriptions that will help most of those patients whose moment-in-care falls into a common grouping. An example of a moment-in-care hierarchy is shown in Table 5.1 on pages 80 and 81. These groupings can provide some degree of specificity.

Table 5.1 Moments in Care for Congestive Heart Failure

Triggering Information (what the system knows)	Moment in Care
Self-awareness of symptoms	**1.0 Prediagnosis** (symptoms, concerns, choosing a physician, first visit prep)
Reason for visit: symptom (shortness of breath)	**1.3 Preparing for Visit** (shortness of breath)
Clinician prescription Positive test results First visit with CHF-ICD-9 diagnosis	**2.0 Initial Treatment**
EMR, medication order, etc.	**2.1 Prescription of Medication** Specific medication would be identified as a clinical qualifier.
Clinician Ix prescription on first diagnosis First diagnosis noted by billing system	**2.3 Home Treatment**
Clinician prescription—based on symptoms Nurse call center prescription—based on symptoms System prescription—based on medical test results	**3.0 Ongoing Medical Concerns** (worsening, complications, hospital admission, etc.) Information prescription fine-tuned by clinical qualifiers of orders such as Bypass, Angioplasty, Transplant, etc.
Clinician prescription Self-prescription EMR Scheduling system—with a reason for visit of CHF (system-generated prescriptions can be time-phased for periodic delivery)	**4.0 Living With Congestive Heart Failure (CHF)**
Clinician prescription Self-prescription System-generated based on hospitalization and prior patient preference assessment	**5.0 End-of-Life Care With CHF** (palliative options)

Consumer Questions Within the Moment of Care

- What is heart failure? What are the symptoms? What might happen?
- Should I seek care? How do I choose a doctor?

- How do I prepare for a visit to diagnose my shortness of breath?

- What causes CHF? What type do I have?
- What's my prognosis? Is CHF reversible?
- What should I do first?

- Do I need this medication?
- What does it do? What are its benefits and side effects?
- Did I get the right medication and dose?
- What if I miss a dose or stop taking it?

- How do I limit salt?
- What should I eat?
- How much should I exercise? How much rest do I need?
- How can I avoid colds and the flu?

- Do I need hospitalization? How do I prepare to go?
- Do I need surgery?
- Do I need different medications?
- How do I get better and avoid hospitalization?
- What should I do when I return from the hospital?

- What lifestyle changes should I make?
- Why do I need to monitor my weight?
- How often should I see my doctor?
- How do people die of CHF? Do I need to write a living will?
- What are the guidelines for medications, salt, fluids, exercise, weight, and smoking?

- What are the options for care near the end of life?
- How does a family prepare for a CHF death?

Clinical Qualifiers: Tuning In to Clinical Findings

Clinical qualifiers can also be used to target the information prescription with even more precision. Clinical qualifiers are medical facts known about the patient or the treatment plan that go beyond the moment in care. Clinical qualifiers fall in at least three categories:

- Diagnosis refinements—cause of condition (for example, CHF due to coronary artery disease), type of condition (for example, systolic heart failure rather than diastolic), severity of condition (usually as rated on an objective scale)

- Relevant patient characteristics—age, sex, race

- Co-morbidity characteristics

During a clinic visit with a patient, clinicians consider all of these factors in determining what information would be of most value to that particular patient. While the use of clinical qualifiers is not essential for many Ix applications, some uses of automated information prescriptions will require the capture and use of some or all of these qualifiers before clinically acceptable prescriptions can be delivered.

Balancing Precision and Efficiency

Precision needs to be balanced against efficiency. The more closely an information prescription can be designed around the precise moment in care that the patient is facing, the more valuable and appreciated the information will be. However, the value gained in defining the moment in care with increased precision must be balanced against the added cost and complexity that level of precision requires. Information prescriptions that more precisely describe a patient's clinical reality but have little impact on the treatment options or decisions that the patient faces may not be worth the added cost of developing, updating, and administering them.

The need for efficiency highlights one of the major challenges of system-prescribed information therapy: how to use existing information sources to predict, with as much accuracy and precision as possible, which moment in care the individual is in. That challenge is met with information triggers.

Information Triggers

Information triggers are data elements that predict a moment in care. When data that matches a preset pattern is captured and stored within existing information systems, it can automatically trigger an information prescription. Information triggers can be found in every aspect of medical care: visit prep, billing, testing, medication, preauthorization, and preventive services.

Appointment Request Triggers

One of the most straightforward uses of information therapy is sending an information prescription to help a person prepare for a clinic visit. All that is needed to implement an effective application is knowledge of the reason for a visit and the patient's secure e-mail address. The "reason for visit" becomes the primary trigger. The moment in care becomes "Preparing for a clinic visit for ____." (Of course, other information triggers can help to refine the moment in care, which would allow for a more precise and more helpful information prescription.)

Types of Triggers

- *Appointment request*
- *Billing*
- *Testing*
- *Medications*
- *Preauthorization*
- *Preventive services*

Example 4
Susan Morrison

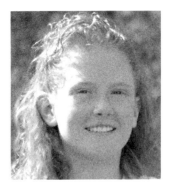

Ix Prescription from Dr. Wood's Clinic

Trigger: Call for appointment

Reason for Visit: Wrist injury

Moments in Care:
- Preparing for visit, wrist pain/injury
- TD booster—due

Patient: Susan Morrison (age 12)

Ix Recipient: Mary Morrison (mother)

Situation: Susan injured her wrist in a basketball game. When Mary called Dr. Wood's office to schedule an appointment, the appointments clerk entered the term "wrist injury" in the clinic's scheduling software as the "reason for visit."

The clinic's Ix system used that information to predict that Susan was at a moment in care described as "wrist pain: prediagnosis." The clinic's Ix system had previously linked that moment in care for all patients to information on "home treatment for finger, hand, and wrist injuries" and "how to prepare for a visit about finger, hand and wrist injuries."

Ix Action: By the end of Mary's call, the Ix system had already placed links to the key information in a secure messaging system under Susan's file and sent Mrs. Morrison an e-mail encouraging her to review it. (The e-mail may also be sent directly to Susan, if desired.)

Because the messaging was done automatically, the scheduling clerk did not need to take any extra steps other than to alert Mrs. Morrison that she may be receiving the information prescription.

The system also notes that there is no record that Susan has had a tetanus/diphtheria booster and adds a routine immunization scheduling message.

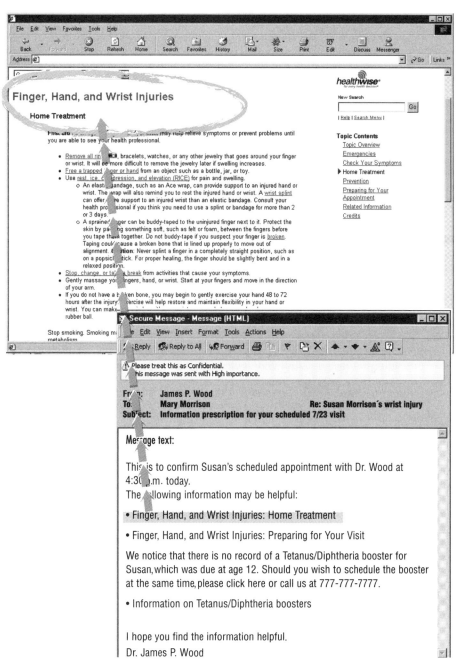

Finger, Hand, and Wrist Injuries

Home Treatment

First aid ... may help relieve symptoms or prevent problems until you are able to see your health professional.

- Remove all rings, bracelets, watches, or any other jewelry that goes around your finger or wrist. It will be more difficult to remove the jewelry later if swelling increases.
- Free a trapped finger or hand from an object such as a bottle, jar, or toy.
- Use rest, ice, compression, and elevation (RICE) for pain and swelling.
  - An elastic bandage, such as an Ace wrap, can provide support to an injured hand or wrist. The wrap will also remind you to rest the injured hand or wrist. A wrist splint can offer more support to an injured wrist than an elastic bandage. Consult your health professional if you think you need to use a splint or bandage for more than 2 or 3 days.
  - A sprained finger can be buddy-taped to the uninjured finger next to it. Protect the skin by padding something soft, such as felt or foam, between the fingers before you tape them together. Do not buddy-tape if you suspect your finger is broken. Taping could cause a broken bone that is lined up properly to move out of alignment. Caution: Never splint a finger in a completely straight position, such as on a popsicle stick. For proper healing, the finger should be slightly bent and in a relaxed position.
- Stop, change, or take a break from activities that cause your symptoms.
- Gently massage your fingers, hand, or wrist. Start at your fingers and move in the direction of your arm.
- If you do not have a broken bone, you may begin to gently exercise your hand 48 to 72 hours after the injury. Exercise will help restore and maintain flexibility in your hand or wrist. You can make ... rubber ball.

Stop smoking. Smoking ... metabolism

healthwise®
for every health decision®

New Search
[_____] Go

| Help | Search Menu |

Topic Contents
Topic Overview
Emergencies
Check Your Symptoms
▶ Home Treatment
Prevention
Preparing for Your Appointment
Related Information
Credits

Secure Message - Message [HTML]

File Edit View Insert Format Tools Actions Help

Reply | Reply to All | Forward

⚠ Please treat this as Confidential.
This message was sent with High importance.

From: James P. Wood
To: Mary Morrison   **Re: Susan Morrison's wrist injury**
Subject: Information prescription for your scheduled 7/23 visit

Message text:

This is to confirm Susan's scheduled appointment with Dr. Wood at 4:30 p.m. today.
The following information may be helpful:

• Finger, Hand, and Wrist Injuries: Home Treatment

• Finger, Hand, and Wrist Injuries: Preparing for Your Visit

We notice that there is no record of a Tetanus/Diphtheria booster for Susan, which was due at age 12. Should you wish to schedule the booster at the same time, please click here or call us at 777-777-7777.

• Information on Tetanus/Diphtheria boosters

I hope you find the information helpful.
Dr. James P. Wood

Example 4
To see an example of how this will work, go to
www.informationtherapy.org/examples·

85

Example:

When Mary Morrison's 12-year-old daughter, Susan, injured her wrist in a basketball game, Mary called Dr. Wood's office to schedule an appointment. The appointments clerk at the clinic entered the term "wrist pain—injury" in the clinic's scheduling software as the "reason for visit." The clinic's Ix system used that information to predict that Susan was at a moment in care described as "wrist pain: prediagnosis." The clinic's Ix system had previously linked that moment in care for all patients to information on "home treatment for finger, hand, and wrist injuries" and "how to prepare for a visit about finger, hand, and wrist injuries."

By the end of Mary's call, the Ix system would have already placed links to the key information in a secure messaging system under Susan's file and sent Mrs. Morrison an e-mail encouraging her to review it. (The e-mail may also be sent directly to Susan.) Because the messaging was done automatically, the scheduling clerk did not need to take any extra steps other than to alert Mrs. Morrison that she may be receiving the information prescription.

In this case, the home treatment for wrist pain is fairly simple. The information would convey to Susan the need to take off any rings before swelling in the hand made removal difficult. RICE instructions (rest, ice, compression, and elevation) and general guidelines for use of a nonaspirin pain reliever would also be helpful.

In a simple system, Susan and Mary Morrison would get the same information prescription as any other person calling to schedule a "wrist pain" appointment. However, as information systems mature, other information known about Susan could be used to more finely hone the prescription to Susan's particular needs. In a mature system, Susan might well get a different set of home treatment guidelines than would her grandmother, Lori, age 73, if Lori had called for a wrist pain appointment.

Susan might also get additional information about health issues that are unrelated to the wrist pain. For example, if the clinic's information systems included an electronic medical record, the information prescriptions might also include a note that Susan was due for a tetanus booster. A simple one-click confirmation could arrange for the additional service during the wrist pain visit.

It may also be that Susan's wrist sprain is minor and needs only good home treatment and watchful waiting for a few days or weeks. The information prescription could include a link to interactive self-triage information that would allow Mary and Susan to judge whether the visit was really needed. If self-care is appropriate, they could call back to cancel the appointment or to change it to one for the tetanus booster only.

Billing System Triggers

In some cases a health plan's or clinic system's knowledge about a patient may be limited to what is transmitted in billing records. Alas, this is not necessarily the best place to begin, but it can be done. There are at least two inherent problems with using a billing system's data to predict a moment in care. First, the coding system is designed as a reimbursement tool, not as a tool to denote moments in care. This leads to coding inaccuracies. And second, the timing is dubious.

Accuracy and precision are real bugbears; some physicians and clinics place little emphasis on using accurate codes. When the codes are used for reimbursement only, there is no clinical incentive to enter a specific diagnosis code when a general, easy-to-remember code will result in the same payment. The coding is done by an office support person who interprets what the coding should be based upon the chart. These interpretations can lead to misinterpretations and inaccuracies.

Coding is also usually done to a general level and can include all diseases touched upon, not just the one that specifically needs the prescription information. For example, a patient can come in with diabetes that is not very well controlled. The doctor may also determine that the patient's lipid picture does not look good. Plus, the patient's blood pressure is checked to make sure that her hypertension is controlled. The billing coding for that particular visit could well include diabetes, hyperlipidemia, and hypertension. Just what, then, is the moment in care?

Example 5
Jane Williams

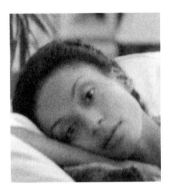

Ix Prescription from XYZ Health Plan

Trigger: Billing for visit

Diagnosis Recorded: Hashimoto's thyroiditis: ICD-9 245.2

Moments in Care:

Hashimoto's thyroiditis: Early treatment

Patient: Jane Williams

Situation: Jackson Williams' daughter, Jane, visited her family physician because she had been feeling tired and without energy for months.

During the exam, Dr. Judith Clark discovered that, in addition to her tiredness and her low spirits, Jane had a palpable but painless lump on the front of her throat.

After appropriate testing, Dr. Clark established the diagnosis of Hypothyroidism—Hashimoto's thyroiditis. The ICD-9 code (245.2) was included in the electronic billing of the visit to Jane's health plan, XYZ Health.

Ix Action: XYZ Health's data warehouse immediately shared the information with XYZ's information therapy system. Because this was the first time that the code had been used for a service Jane received, her moment in care was classified as Hashimoto's thyroiditis: Early treatment.

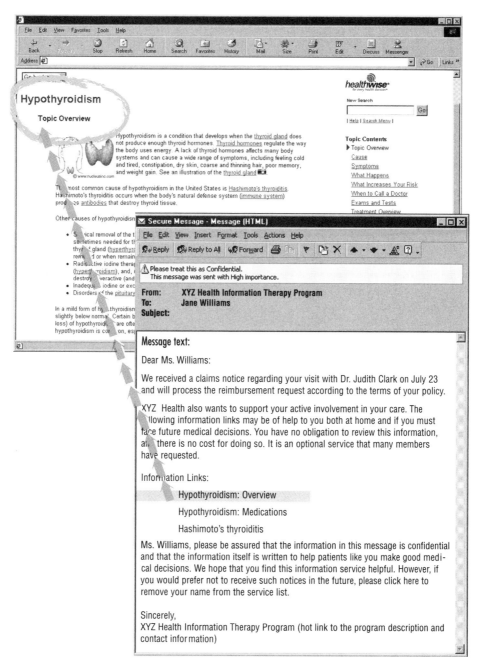

Hypothyroidism

Topic Overview

Hypothyroidism is a condition that develops when the thyroid gland does not produce enough thyroid hormones. Thyroid hormones regulate the way the body uses energy. A lack of thyroid hormones affects many body systems and can cause a wide range of symptoms, including feeling dull and tired, constipation, dry skin, coarse and thinning hair, poor memory, and weight gain. See an illustration of the thyroid gland.

The most common cause of hypothyroidism in the United States is Hashimoto's thyroiditis. Hashimoto's thyroiditis occurs when the body's natural defense system (immune system) produces antibodies that destroy thyroid tissue.

Other causes of hypothyroidism

- Surgical removal of the thyroid, sometimes needed for thyroid gland (hyperthyroidism removed or when remaining
- Radioactive iodine therapy (hyperthyroidism), and destroy overactive (and
- Inadequate iodine or excess
- Disorders of the pituitary

In a mild form of hypothyroidism slightly below normal. Certain b loss) of hypothyroidism are ofte hypothyroidism is common, es

healthwise
for every health decision

New Search
[Go]

| Help | Search Menu |

Topic Contents
▶ Topic Overview
Cause
Symptoms
What Happens
What Increases Your Risk
When to Call a Doctor
Exams and Tests
Treatment Overview

Secure Message - Message (HTML)

File Edit View Insert Format Tools Actions Help

Reply   Reply to All   Forward

⚠ Please treat this as Confidential.
This message was sent with High importance.

From: XYZ Health Information Therapy Program
To: Jane Williams
Subject:

Message text:

Dear Ms. Williams:

We received a claims notice regarding your visit with Dr. Judith Clark on July 23 and will process the reimbursement request according to the terms of your policy.

XYZ Health also wants to support your active involvement in your care. The following information links may be of help to you both at home and if you must face future medical decisions. You have no obligation to review this information, and there is no cost for doing so. It is an optional service that many members have requested.

Information Links:

    Hypothyroidism: Overview

    Hypothyroidism: Medications

    Hashimoto's thyroiditis

Ms. Williams, please be assured that the information in this message is confidential and that the information itself is written to help patients like you make good medical decisions. We hope that you find this information service helpful. However, if you would prefer not to receive such notices in the future, please click here to remove your name from the service list.

Sincerely,
XYZ Health Information Therapy Program (hot link to the program description and contact information)

Example 5

To see an example of how this will work, go to
www.informationtherapy.org/examples.

The second problem with billing and claims data is timing. If a claim is used to automatically generate an information prescription but the claim is not submitted at the same time that the service is performed, the resulting information prescription may arrive after the moment in care has passed.

A reality check: While the quality of billing information is notoriously poor, it can still be used to trigger information to be sent to patients. At an absolute minimum, a billing transaction lets you know that a specific patient was seen in the clinic on a certain day. That alone is enough to send patients a link to the clinic's Web site with general directions to look up anything that might be concerning them following the visit. It's a minimal intervention, but the invitation may be all that is needed to get the patient engaged and involved in active self-management of a health condition.

In many cases, the billing information will include a diagnosis code that identifies the general area of medical concern the patient is facing. The Ix system could then send the patient a message recognizing the visit and pointing to a menu of topics that might relate to his or her medical concerns. The patient would then select from within the menu the health problem and moment in care that he or she thinks best fits the situation. (In clinics that maintain a high level of discipline and training in the use of diagnostic codes, the billing record can be used to send the patient a message much more targeted to his or her specific problem.)

Again, the more that is known and the greater the confidence in the quality of the information, the more precisely the moment in care can be predicted.

Using Billing System Codes to Trigger Preventive Services

Health organizations can also use billing system triggers in focused improvement efforts around a specific illness. Perhaps a health plan's HEDIS® (Health Plan Employer Data and Information Set) report had shown that its diabetic members have a worse-than-average record of blood sugar control and retinal exams. The Ix system could send periodic eye exam reminders and invitations to see an eye care professional to all patients with clinic visits in the past year that had a diagnosis code indicating diabetes. The reminders and invitations would include links to self-care guidelines on how to eat appropriately and manage blood sugar well.

Using data mining methods, health plans and clinics can search on any number of parameters to identify and target a specific group of members or patients who might benefit from a particular "information set." Targeted claims-based programs can start small with only a few targeted diagnoses and later grow to include more high-cost and high-risk conditions.

Test-Reporting Triggers

Test-reporting triggers can be used by the doctor who orders the test, the testing organization that reports the information to the doctor, or the health plan that gets notification that the test was performed.

These applications are becoming easier with the rapid development of automated test-reporting systems. These systems notify the physician (and sometimes the patient) of test results as soon as the results are known. These systems have all the information needed to launch a basic Ix prescription: patient name, name of test, result of test, and, often, patient diagnosis.

Consider the ubiquitous cholesterol test and report. When a clinic received the results of a cholesterol test, it could automatically send the patient a summary of the report and an information prescription on how to understand the test results. If a physician preferred to withhold the results until he or she could go over them with the patient in person, the clinic could at least send an explanation of the test so that the patient could better understand the explanation at the next visit.

Of course, it might have been even better for the clinic to have sent such an explanation at the time the test was ordered. Knowledge about how to prepare in advance of the test can help to prevent inaccurate results and the need for retesting.

Example 6
Jack Morrison

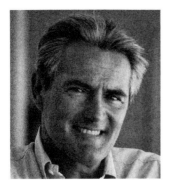

Ix Prescription from Dr. Wood's Clinic

Trigger: Lab report

Type of Test:
LDL/HDL/Total
Cholesterol

Results:
LDL: 162
HDL: 45
Total: 239

Moments in Care:

Cholesterol test
results: Moderate to
high

Patient: Jack Morrison

Situation: At a recent checkup, Dr. Wood did a cholesterol test on Jack Morrison, Mary's husband. Several days later, Jack got a call from Dr. Wood's nurse saying that the results were back and that his scores were as follows:

- LDL Cholesterol: 162 mg/dL (milligrams per deciliter)
- HDL Cholesterol: 45 mg/dL
- Total Cholesterol: 239 mg/dL

Jack wrote down the numbers and remembered the nurse saying that the results were "not too bad" but that he might want to watch what he eats.

Ix Action: In addition to the nurse call, Dr. Wood's clinic sent him a notice of a secure message prepared automatically by their information therapy system based on the CPT numbers 83718 and 83721 associated with the cholesterol testing. The Ix system associated this information with the moment in care "Cholesterol test results— Moderate to High."

The Ix system instantaneously sent Jack an e-mail directing him to the XYZ secure messaging system. After instant authentication, Jack reached the message shown on the next page.

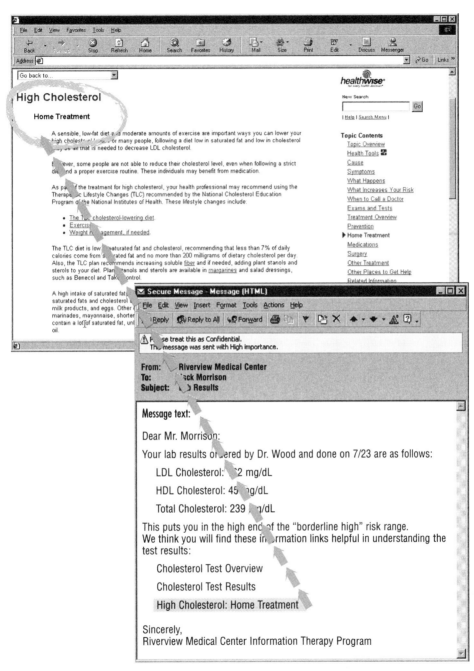

High Cholesterol

Home Treatment

A sensible, low-fat diet and moderate amounts of exercise are important ways you can lower your high cholesterol level. For many people, following a diet low in saturated fat and low in cholesterol may be all that is needed to decrease LDL cholesterol.

However, some people are not able to reduce their cholesterol level, even when following a strict diet and a proper exercise routine. These individuals may benefit from medication.

As part of the treatment for high cholesterol, your health professional may recommend using the Therapeutic Lifestyle Changes (TLC) recommended by the National Cholesterol Education Program of the National Institutes of Health. These lifestyle changes include:

- The TLC cholesterol-lowering diet.
- Exercise.
- Weight management, if needed.

The TLC diet is low in saturated fat and cholesterol, recommending that less than 7% of daily calories come from saturated fat and no more than 200 milligrams of dietary cholesterol per day. Also, the TLC plan recommends increasing soluble fiber and if needed, adding plant stanols and sterols to your diet. Plant stanols and sterols are available in margarines and salad dressings, such as Benecol and Take Control.

A high intake of saturated fats... saturated fats and cholesterol... milk products, and eggs. Other... marinades, mayonnaise, shorten... contain a lot of saturated fat, unl... oil.

healthwise®

New Search

[Help | Search Menu]

Topic Contents
Topic Overview
Health Tools
Cause
Symptoms
What Happens
What Increases Your Risk
When to Call a Doctor
Exams and Tests
Treatment Overview
Prevention
▶ Home Treatment
Medications
Surgery
Other Treatment
Other Places to Get Help
Related Information

Secure Message - Message (HTML)

⚠ Please treat this as Confidential.
The message was sent with High importance.

From: Riverview Medical Center
To: Jack Morrison
Subject: Lab Results

Message text:

Dear Mr. Morrison:

Your lab results ordered by Dr. Wood and done on 7/23 are as follows:

    LDL Cholesterol: 2 mg/dL

    HDL Cholesterol: 45 mg/dL

    Total Cholesterol: 239 mg/dL

This puts you in the high end of the "borderline high" risk range.
We think you will find these information links helpful in understanding the test results:

    Cholesterol Test Overview

    Cholesterol Test Results

    High Cholesterol: Home Treatment

Sincerely,
Riverview Medical Center Information Therapy Program

Example 6

To see an example of how this will work, go to
www.informationtherapy.org/examples.

Medication Order Triggers

Medication prescriptions provide a ready supply of triggers for related information prescriptions. Every new medication prescribed to patients should come with information: the medication's name, dose, frequency of dose, reason for prescription, how it works, what it looks like, how to take it, contraindications, and possible side effects. Paired with the general information that pharmacies provide, this type of information prescription is an additional safeguard against medication errors. It also promotes safer and more effective use of medications.

Medication orders can also be predictive of broader moments in care. The first prescription of insulin for a 9-year-old, for example, may predict a moment in care described by "Early diagnosis and treatment of diabetes." Similarly, the first prescription of Prozac could be used to send the patient links to depression-related information. The list of possibilities is extensive.

The rapid development of computerized order entry and electronic medical records systems in clinics and hospitals bodes well for the use of medication orders as information triggers. Once the system has the patient and medication information for the drug prescription, the information prescription can be suggested, selected, and sent with just two taps on a clinician's PDA (personal digital assistant) or by an automatic algorithm of the Ix system.

Preauthorization Triggers

Another rich source of information triggers are the preauthorizations that many insurers and managed care plans require before major procedures or hospitalizations—some of the most financially and medically important moments in care. These systems already contain all of the information needed to judge whether the requested service will be covered by the plan. It is relatively easy to use that same information to trigger an information prescription. The trigger source (preauthorization) plus the diagnosis can combine to identify a very specific description of a moment in care.

In some cases, the individual who receives such information may change his or her mind about the surgery. The goal of the information prescription is improved understanding and active, informed consent.

The information should noticeably reduce the number who say about surgery, "I wouldn't have done it if I had known this was likely to happen." The information can help assure that patients will be satisfied with their treatment experiences.

Preventive Service Triggers

Many different information triggers can be used to send a person information about disease prevention. The goal is to encourage healthy behavior or promote a preventive service by sending the right preventive message to the right person at the right time. The simplest systems use birth dates to trigger birthday reminders about periodic preventive services that are recommended on an annual or semiannual basis. The more that is known about the individual, however, the more specific the information prescription can be. Sophisticated systems with richer databases can combine moments in care with clinical qualifiers, as discussed on page 82, to create more precisely targeted information prescriptions.

Preventive message triggers might also come from other, unrelated information. For example, the scheduling of a child's clinic visit for a cold or other acute illness could trigger an information prescription about getting immunizations up to date at the same time.

Not all prevention message triggers need to come directly from individual patient data. Reports of high pollen counts can be used to trigger messages for allergy sufferers. Likewise, heat waves, cold spells, mosquito season, sunburn season, and other periodic high-risk situations can be combined with more basic information about patients to trigger targeted messages. Because mass e-mailing can result in many calls to the clinic or even scheduled appointments for related issues, it may be smart to stagger such messages over a few days or weeks.

Example 7
Mary Morrison

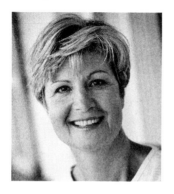

Ix Prescription from AAA PBM

Trigger: Prescription order from James P. Wood, MD

Medication: Lamisil (terbinafine) NDC 0078-0179-05

Moments in Care:

Medication prescription

Patient: Mary Morrison

Situation: Mary suffers from fungal infections in her toenails. She received a prescription of terbinafine (Lamisil), an antifungal medication, from Dr. Wood during a recent visit.

She filled the prescription at a local drugstore.

Ix Action: A record of the prescription was automatically sent to the AAA Pharmacy Benefits Management company that contracts with XYZ Health to monitor and manage her prescriptions. The record included the following information:

Name and ID Number: Mary Morrison, 3456789012

Diagnosis: ICD-9 110.1 (Toenail Fungus Infection)

Medication Ordered: NDC 0078-0179-05 (Lamisil (terbinafine))

Treating Physician: Provider Number 98765 (Dr. James P. Wood)

AAA's information therapy system checked to see if Mary had received the same prescription before. It instantaneously sent Mary an e-mail directing her to the AAA secure messaging system. After instant authentication, Mary reached the message shown on the next page.

Mary also suffers from occasional heartburn. Heartburn is sometimes treated with the drug cimetidine (Tagamet). However, terbinafine and cimetidine are incompatible drugs; taken together, they can cause serious side effects. If Mary had been prescribed cimetidine by another doctor and not mentioned it to Dr. Wood, it is possible that she would have a serious problem. Giving her complete medication information provides one more safeguard against a potentially serious medical mistake.

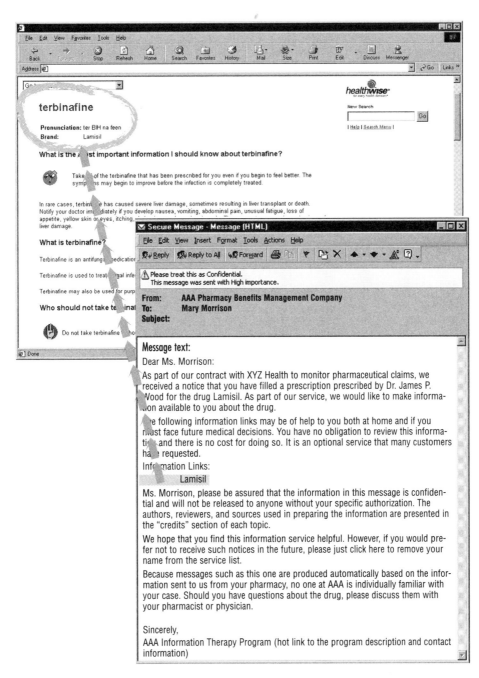

terbinafine

Pronunciation: ter BIH na feen
Brand: Lamisil

What is the most important information I should know about terbinafine?

Take all of the terbinafine that has been prescribed for you even if you begin to feel better. The symptoms may begin to improve before the infection is completely treated.

In rare cases, terbinafine has caused severe liver damage, sometimes resulting in liver transplant or death. Notify your doctor immediately if you develop nausea, vomiting, abdominal pain, unusual fatigue, loss of appetite, yellow skin or eyes, itching, liver damage.

What is terbinafine?

Terbinafine is an antifungal medication

Terbinafine is used to treat fungal infe

Terbinafine may also be used for purp

Who should not take terbinal

Do not take terbinafine who

healthwise®
for every health decision®

New Search

[Help | Search Menu]

Secure Message - Message [HTML]

File Edit View Insert Format Tools Actions Help

Reply   Reply to All   Forward

Please treat this as Confidential.
This message was sent with High importance.

From: AAA Pharmacy Benefits Management Company
To: Mary Morrison
Subject:

Message text:

Dear Ms. Morrison:

As part of our contract with XYZ Health to monitor pharmaceutical claims, we received a notice that you have filled a prescription prescribed by Dr. James P. Wood for the drug Lamisil. As part of our service, we would like to make information available to you about the drug.

The following information links may be of help to you both at home and if you must face future medical decisions. You have no obligation to review this information and there is no cost for doing so. It is an optional service that many customers have requested.

Information Links:

    Lamisil

Ms. Morrison, please be assured that the information in this message is confidential and will not be released to anyone without your specific authorization. The authors, reviewers, and sources used in preparing the information are presented in the "credits" section of each topic.

We hope that you find this information service helpful. However, if you would prefer not to receive such notices in the future, please just click here to remove your name from the service list.

Because messages such as this one are produced automatically based on the information sent to us from your pharmacy, no one at AAA is individually familiar with your case. Should you have questions about the drug, please discuss them with your pharmacist or physician.

Sincerely,

AAA Information Therapy Program (hot link to the program description and contact information)

Example 7

To see an example of how this will work, go to
www.informationtherapy.org/examples.

Example 8
Jackson Williams

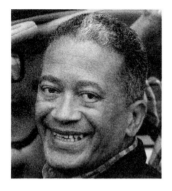

Ix Prescription from ABC Health Plan

Trigger: Surgery preauthorization

Moments in Care:
- Preparing for surgery
- Preparing for hospitalization

Patient: Jackson Williams

Situation: Jackson visited urologist Raymond Crane to consider surgery. After the exam and a review of the treatment options, Jackson decided to proceed with the urologist's recommendation for a TURP (transurethral resection of the prostate). Dr. Crane's office then called ABC Health Plan for authorization to proceed with the surgery, which was approved.

Name and ID Number: Jackson Williams, 135791

Diagnosis: ICD-9 600.0 (BPH, Benign prostatic hyperplasia)

Procedure Authorization: CPT 52601 (TURP)

Physician: Provider Number 89765 (Dr. Raymond J. Crane)

Status: Approved

Ix Action: ABC's information therapy system accessed the preauthorization information, assigned Jackson to the moment in care of "Preparing for hospitalization and surgery for TURP," and sent the corresponding Ix prescription.

The information prescription includes detailed information on the surgical risks and the alternatives to surgical treatment that is required for informed consent. At the health plan's option, the message can highlight a decision guide about whether or not to have surgery for an enlarged prostate. Jackson can use the information to better understand the surgery and to prepare for the hospitalization and his recovery period. Or he may rethink his options.

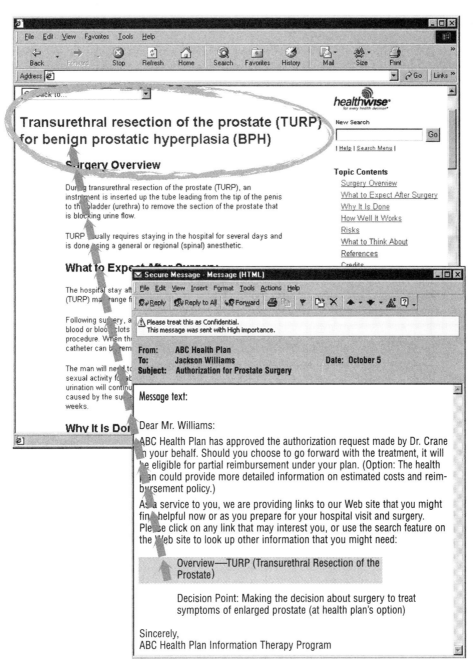

File   Edit   View   Favorites   Tools   Help

Back   Forward   Stop   Refresh   Home   Search   Favorites   History   Mail   Size   Print

Address

Go   Links »

Go back to...

healthwise·
for every health decision·

Transurethral resection of the prostate (TURP) for benign prostatic hyperplasia (BPH)

New Search

Go

| Help | Search Menu |

Surgery Overview

During transurethral resection of the prostate (TURP), an instrument is inserted up the tube leading from the tip of the penis to the bladder (urethra) to remove the section of the prostate that is blocking urine flow.

TURP usually requires staying in the hospital for several days and is done using a general or regional (spinal) anesthetic.

Topic Contents
Surgery Overview
What to Expect After Surgery
Why It Is Done
How Well It Works
Risks
What to Think About
References
Credits

What to Expect After Surgery

The hospital stay after (TURP) may range fi

Following surgery, a blood or blood clots procedure. When th catheter can be rem

The man will need to sexual activity for ab urination will continu caused by the su weeks.

Why It Is Done

Secure Message - Message (HTML)

File   Edit   View   Insert   Format   Tools   Actions   Help

Reply   Reply to All   Forward

⚠ Please treat this as Confidential.
This message was sent with High importance.

From: ABC Health Plan
To: Jackson Williams   Date: October 5
Subject: Authorization for Prostate Surgery

Message text:

Dear Mr. Williams:

ABC Health Plan has approved the authorization request made by Dr. Crane on your behalf. Should you choose to go forward with the treatment, it will be eligible for partial reimbursement under your plan. (Option: The health plan could provide more detailed information on estimated costs and reimbursement policy.)

As a service to you, we are providing links to our Web site that you might find helpful now or as you prepare for your hospital visit and surgery. Please click on any link that may interest you, or use the search feature on the Web site to look up other information that you might need:

Overview—TURP (Transurethral Resection of the Prostate)

Decision Point: Making the decision about surgery to treat symptoms of enlarged prostate (at health plan's option)

Sincerely,
ABC Health Plan Information Therapy Program

Example 8

To see an example of how this will work, go to
www.informationtherapy.org/examples.

Delivering the Message

In addition to presenting links to the "right information to the right person at the right time," each information prescription should include a message designed to accomplish three things:

1. **Personalization.** The message must personalize the information prescription so that the recipient knows that it is indeed meant for him or her.

2. **Explanation.** The message must tell the recipient why he or she is getting the information prescription.

3. **Motivation.** The message must motivate and encourage the recipient to follow the links and to review the information that might lead to a better health decision or better health.

Personalization is accomplished by correctly using the person's name in the opening of the message. Keeping track of how a patient or member wishes to be addressed is important. Use of the right name can help open the mind's door just as easily as using the wrong name can close it. The message should convey the impression that it is, indeed, designed especially for the recipient.

Explanation is also important—Why me? Why now? Why this? The better an individual understands the reason why he or she is getting a particular message, the more likely he or she will act on it. When possible, the message should be linked to a recent or scheduled clinical event like an office visit, lab test, or hospitalization. People are more likely to accept and use information that is sent as an extension of a medical service. The explanation should also quell any fears that would otherwise be raised over privacy. Since personalized health information is obviously used in preparing the information prescription, it is essential to give assurance that the use is appropriate and that the information will not be provided to any third party or person not authorized by the individual through prior agreement.

The motivational power of system-prescribed information may never be as great as that of information coming directly from the patient's health professional. But system-generated messages can be more effective when they motivate a person toward a call to action. Messages that suggest an expectation of the patient's review of the information without implying that it is an absolute requirement also work well.

The nature of the message depends greatly on the trigger source as well as the trigger. The identification of a diagnosis from a billing code may be much less precise than one gained from a preauthorization request. When the trigger source is precise, the call to action can be relatively directive—if not toward treatment, then toward the review of information about treatment options. When the information source is less reliable or precise, the call to action must be adjusted accordingly. Sometimes the only "call" is for the patient to assess whether any of the information links are of interest.

Tailored Messaging: Up Close and Even More Personal

In delivering messages to consumers, there's personal, there's targeted, and then there's tailored.

A personalized health message, at its most basic, uses the consumer's name and sends that person general health information: "Dear Sue: Congratulations on your pregnancy. Here is a list of recommended second trimester exams and tests . . ."

A targeted health message does further refinement: "Dear Sue: Congratulations on your pregnancy. Because this is your first pregnancy and you are over age 35, we would like to draw your attention to . . ."

A tailored health message goes beyond that by approximating a personal care-counseling session: "Dear Sue: Congratulations on your pregnancy. Because this is your first pregnancy and you are over age 35 and have special concerns about your vegetarian diet, we would like to bring to your special attention . . ." Tailored messages can be made to order by using words or images identified by Sue to be particularly motivating.

Tailored messaging has been shown to increase motivational effectiveness, promote and support behavioral change, and improve medical outcomes.[4] So how is it possible to get at that level of specificity? Tailoring systems use detailed questionnaires and assessments, based upon health communication and behavioral science theory, to gather information about an individual's health behaviors, attitudes and beliefs, motivations, family situation, readiness for change, and preferred learning styles. Once a system has that kind of information about the person, messages to that person can be honed for maximum effectiveness. Tailored messaging is, in effect, reaching the ultimate target of one.

Current uses of tailored messaging are primarily limited to behavioral change programs around lifestyle issues such as smoking, fitness, nutrition, and stress management. Current uses of information therapy, in contrast, are hinged upon a specific moment in care. Eventually, the same technology employed by tailoring systems can be used to tailor similar messages for more specific elements of disease self-management or decision support. In the future, tailored Ix messaging will become the gold standard.

More about tailored messaging is presented in the profile on HealthMedia, Inc. on page 179.

Blocking Factors: When Not to Send a Message

Anytime information is selected and sent automatically, as with system-prescribed information, there are risks. The wrong information might go out. The wrong person might be notified. The information might go out at the wrong time. One way to reduce the chance of inappropriate message delivery is to identify and assign blocking factors to messages associated with each moment in care.

A blocking factor is an identifiable condition that would prevent the sending of a message. Blocking factors can be age, sex, previous service, a medical condition, or health status related and specific to a health organization's guidelines. Blocking factors include:

• Gender appropriateness: Don't send an information prescription on PSA prostate tests to a woman (unless you are specifically trying to engage women to reinforce a message for their spouses).

- Age appropriateness: Don't send an information prescription on smoking cessation to a 2-year-old.

- Service appropriateness: Don't send a reminder message for immunizations if the records show no immunization is due.

- Medical condition appropriateness: Don't send Pap test reminders to women who have had a hysterectomy for noncancerous reasons.

- Health status appropriateness: Don't send a message to any patient who is no longer living.

- Organization-specific appropriateness: A Catholic hospital may choose not to send information related to birth control or abortion.

The use of blocking factors within Ix programs will help all those involved gain confidence that they will not be embarrassed by sending messages that are obviously inappropriate.

Technical Notes: The Language of Triggers and Intelligent Content

In any automated system, a basic barrier to overcome is the need to standardize all inputs. In information therapy, this is accomplished by using structured medical languages and coding systems to standardize all trigger source information. These codes will become the language of information triggers.

While there are literally scores of structured languages and code sets in use within medical applications today, four common to most U.S.-based health organizations are of particular importance to information therapy: ICD-9 codes, CPT codes, SNOMED®, and NDC. All are described below. Although they clearly overlap, each focuses on a different area of medical information. Because these codes are in common use within existing health information systems, they can be helpful in triggering prescriptions that send the right information to the right person at the right time.

ICD-9: International Classification of Disease, 9th Revision, World Health Organization

ICD-9 is an acronym for International Classification of Disease, 9th Revision. ICD-9 is a statistical classification system that arranges diseases and injuries into groups according to established criteria. Most ICD-9 codes are numeric and consist of three, four, or five numbers and a description. ICD-9 codes are structured with parent- and child-level codes. Parent codes are the three-digit codes that encompass specific diagnoses. The children-level codes are the four- and five-digit codes, below the parent code, that further define the diagnosis related to the disease state. The World Health Organization revises the codes approximately every 10 years. Annual updates are published by the Center for Medicare and Medicaid Services (CMS), formerly HCFA.[5]

CPT®-4: Current Procedural Terminology, Fourth Edition, American Medical Association

Current Procedural Terminology (CPT), Fourth Edition, is a listing of descriptive terms and identifying codes for reporting medical services and procedures performed by physicians. The purpose of CPT is to provide a uniform language that accurately describes medical, surgical, and diagnostic services. The CPT coding schema starts with six broad categories (Evaluation and Management, Anesthesiology, Surgery, Radiology, Pathology/Laboratory, and Medicine). Within these categories, the codes are set out in an order that makes sense for that category. For example, anesthesiology codes are arranged by part of the body (head, neck, thorax, etc.), while medicine codes are arranged generally by specialty (ophthalmology, cardiovascular, pulmonary, etc.). CPT-4 is published annually by the American Medical Association.[6]

SNOMED®: Systematized Nomenclature of Medicine, College of American Pathologists

The Systematized Nomenclature of Medicine is a large and comprehensive multiaxial code system for medical vocabulary. Unlike ICD-9 and CPT-4, SNOMED is not used for billing in the United States. Its system of concepts, concept codes, terms, term codes, and hierarchies is used to represent clinical information and was created for indexing the entire medical record.

SNOMED is used in more than 40 countries and allows for consistent gathering of detailed clinical information, thus enabling providers of various specialties and researchers to share a common understanding across sites of care and computer systems. SNOMED codes and terms enable the retrieval of information for disease management or research performance of outcomes analysis for quality improvement.[7]

NDC: National Drug Code

A fourth coding/language system in common use is the National Drug Code (NDC), which precisely identifies the drug or medication prescribed by a physician to a patient. Because the NDC is used by pharmacists to fill prescriptions, much effort is spent in assuring the accuracy of the code. The NDC can be considered a reliable trigger source for medications. However, because a single medication may be prescribed for many different health problems, medication codes are not always precise indicators of the precise moment in care that the patient faces.

Interface Standards

In addition to the structured languages and codes, several interface standards are being accepted across the health care spectrum. Interface standards enable software to connect one information system to another and seamlessly share data or outputs. By eliminating the need for double entry of common data, they greatly streamline the data collection process for each application involved.

HL7: Health Level Seven, Inc.

Health Level Seven (HL7) is an interface standard for exchanging and transferring health data between computer systems. HL7 controls demographics and other messaging standards. "Level Seven" refers to the application level, which is the highest level of the International Standards Organization's (ISO) communications model for Open Systems Interconnection (OSI). The application level addresses definition of the data to be exchanged, the timing of the interchange, and the communication of certain errors to the application. The seventh level supports such functions as security checks, participant identification, availability checks, exchange mechanism negotiations, and data exchange structuring. HL7 focuses on the interface requirements of the entire health organization.[8]

CCOW: Clinical Context Object Workgroup

Clinical Context Object Workgroup (CCOW), a member of the HL7 organization, has defined the HL7 Context Management Specification as a set of data definitions and system architecture used to maintain clinical context across applications. Clinical context is an information status that a user establishes and modifies while interacting at the point-of-use (e.g., a clinical desktop or personal digital assistant). For example, a hospital may wish to pull information from its billing system, master patient index, X-ray system, lab system, or customer relationship management system as part of its Ix program. Use of the CCOW standard would simplify the technical tasks for integrating all of the pieces to achieve a better information prescription.

CCOW is not a lexicon in the vein of ICD-9, CPT-4, or SNOMED. There are two main components to the CCOW specification: context definitions and context management architecture. Context definitions are used to define a common item shared between applications. Context management architecture is a technology-neutral design for a system that employs the CCOW definitions. The specification defines the applications, interfaces, and business rules that combine to hold the desktop clinical context in sync.[9]

One problem with the use of structured languages and code sets is that they can give a false sense of precision. Because these codes go into great detail to distinguish between slightly different diagnoses or procedures, they can lure an organization into thinking that the codes clearly define a precise moment in care. Unfortunately, the garbage-in, garbage-out theory of data collection and reporting is often hard at work here.

In many clinical settings, ICD-9 codes have been used primarily for billing purposes. Because in most cases the accuracy of the code has had absolutely no consequence for patient care or reimbursement, convenience has often won out over specificity. As a result, most coded diagnoses may fall into a few well-remembered codes. This is not likely to change until technology aids make it easier and faster for the coder to select and enter the right code and until some level of accountability for code accuracy is established. It is important for organizations employing information therapy to understand how precisely these codes are used in each clinic setting and to adjust the precision of their information prescriptions accordingly.

"Intelligent" Content

As with all information prescriptions, the quality of system-prescribed information is directly dependent upon the quality of the information used. When the prescriptions are made automatically, it also becomes critical that the information is selected correctly to fit with the moment in care that the information triggers predict. This is facilitated through the use of "intelligent" content. Intelligent content is medical information that is not only evidence-based and up to date but is also tagged with metadata that can be directly linked to one or more coding languages used in the information triggers. Think of it as very thorough indexing.

When content is tagged and indexed, it facilitates linking specific words or topics to specific diagnoses or procedures codes. For example, an ACL tear (and all its subcomponents) would be linked to all relevant ICD-9, CPT, or SNOMED codes. This level of specificity makes it possible to find or "push" the right information to the patient.

Ix Assessment: Where Should a Hospital or Health Plan Begin?

It can be daunting to realize the breadth of opportunities for information therapy in a hospital or health plan. Every information source provides potential triggering information to help launch, enrich, or redirect an information prescription. Every transaction has some Ix possibility. Like clinics that may wish to start information therapy in areas with "low-hanging fruit" or "killer apps" as described on page 64, hospitals and health plans will do well to conduct a full assessment of Ix opportunities before selecting applications for early implementation.

In addition to the work flow-centered, technology-centered, and patient-centered dimensions of clinic assessments mentioned in Appendix B beginning on page 221, hospitals and health plans may wish to add a fourth dimension: the ever-practical bottom line. Which information prescriptions will best help the business plan or the financial viability of the organization? Applications that have an immediate and strong positive impact on the bottom line or other aspects of the business plan will help create an information therapy beachhead as a foundation upon which other Ix applications can be assembled.

System Innovator: A Group Practice

Palo Alto Medical Foundation is a multispecialty group practice that is implementing information prescriptions across its entire spectrum of medical care.

Palo Alto Medical Foundation
www.pamf.org

The Palo Alto Medical Foundation (PAMF) is a multispecialty group practice that began as a small clinic founded in 1930. Based in Palo Alto, California, with satellites throughout the Bay Area, it has operated as a not-for-profit organization since 1981 and is an affiliate of Sutter Health. PAMF's mission is "to provide and integrate quality health care, health education and biomedical research to improve the health status of our region." PAMF has a long tradition of staying at the leading edge of medical technology. It was an early adopter of the electronic medical record (EMR).

Ix Applications

PAMF is implementing information therapy as a by-product of its use of electronic medical records. At the end of an office-based encounter, patients are given a printout of essential information from the visit, including a list of medications, allergies, orders, patient instructions, and other educational material. Through PAMFOnline, patients can view information from their EMR with links to information therapy. Relevant information is automatically linked to elements in the patients' records, such as their diagnoses, medications, or lab tests. Using PAMFOnline, patients can also request appointments, request prescription renewals, view lab test results, and ask for medical advice through a secure Internet-based application.

Q & A with Paul Tang, MD, chief medical information officer

Q: *What has been the patients' response to PAMF Online?*

A: PAMFOnline has been extremely well received by patients who have signed up for the service. It provides a convenient and reliable alternative to traditional means of communication and offers a self-service way to learn about health issues. Patients trust the information linked from PAMFOnline, knowing that their physician group endorses the information.

Q: *How has PAMF pursued physician acceptance of or support for information therapy?*

A: We are providing a library of information resources that physicians can easily incorporate into patient educational materials provided during a visit or online through PAMFOnline.

Q: *What's next for PAMF Online?*

A: We are exploring options to automatically incorporate informational links in standard text reports so that information therapy can be "attached" to any communication with the patient.

Questions from Clinicians

Q: *If I send information prescriptions to my patients, why is system-prescribed information therapy needed?*

A: It is true that if every physician sent information prescriptions as part of each visit or medical service, there would be much less need for system-prescribed information. Until that day arrives, system-generated prescriptions can help inform patients. Any patient can choose to opt out of system prescriptions if he or she is not in need of further information.

Questions from Consumers

Q: *My health plan operates like a business. How can I trust an information prescription that comes from it?*

A: Read the credits on the information as required by URAC accreditation standards. Health plans have an obligation to tell you who wrote and reviewed the information and to describe any influence that the plan had on the development of the information. If the information comes from a credible source and there is no mention of a health plan's role in modifying the content, you can trust the information to be unbiased.

Q: *My health information is private. I'm worried that my health plan might not use the information in my interest. Can it sell this information to others or use it to increase my premiums?*

A: Again, URAC accreditation standards prevent health Web sites from selling or even giving your personal information to anyone without your clear opt-in approval. Look for the URAC seal.

Q: *If I don't want to receive information prescriptions from my hospital, health plan, or clinic, what can I do?*

A: Information therapy programs should provide an opportunity for anyone to opt out of the program. Once you decline the service, you should not get any further messages unless specifically authorized by your doctor.

Q: *I'd love to get information prescriptions every time I receive a health service, but my physician is not ready to do information therapy. How can I get my health plan to start an information therapy service?*

A: Health plans are often responsive to good ideas from their enrolled members and from their employers. Write a letter to encourage the start of an information therapy program and send a copy to your employer's HR department.

New knowledge is the most valuable commodity on earth.
The more truth we have to work with, the richer we become.
Kurt Vonnegut

6

Consumer-Prescribed Information Therapy

Using particularly vivid imagery, Dr. Roy Schwarz, formerly senior vice president of medical education and science for the American Medical Association, told a reporter: "The trend toward patients' access to medical information was inevitable. It's not going to be reversed unless we burn up the globe."

We'd rather not test his assumption, but we do agree. There is no stopping the consumer's quest for medical information—nor should there be. In this new era of medicine, the patient is a vital and fundamental part of the provider team. To be valuable members of that team, patients need full access to good information about their medical conditions, without restriction and without a professional's prescription.

Without good information, patients are vulnerable to medical mistakes, inappropriate treatment, and the hazards of their own behaviors. With good information, people can become engaged in their health care decisions and health behaviors in ways that result in better health, higher satisfaction, and, often, lower cost.

However, because most consumers are not trained in how to use existing medical systems to find the right information at the right time, prescription-strength content must be made available through systems that are easy to search and understand. Self-prescribed or **consumer-prescribed** information therapy connects the patient with the information either through direct searches (on the Internet or at the library, for instance) or by referral from self-help groups, family members, or friends. To be considered information therapy (Ix), consumer-prescribed information must meet the same three criteria required of the other Ix approaches:

1. **The right information.** The information must be prescription-strength. Assessing information quality is often the most challenging part of consumer-prescribed information therapy.

2. **The right person.** The right person is anyone involved in making or carrying out treatment and behavior decisions. Consumer-prescribed Ix solutions often reflect unique insights into who can help with those decisions—insights that are not available to clinicians or health plans.

3. **The right time.** The information must be sought out or referred to the individual based on information about the moment of care that he or she is in or is approaching. Here, too, the consumer-prescribed approach may have an advantage. The patient is usually the first to know that the moment in care may be changing.

Because no professional is directly involved in consumer-prescribed information therapy, it raises the question of the validity and appropriateness of the information prescriptions. However, the close bonds, trust, and dedicated caring that develop among friends, family, and members of support groups compensate for that risk. With careful review of the information and its source, people can judge for themselves whether the information is something they can trust.

Why Encourage Consumer-Prescribed Information?

For clinicians who have endorsed the importance that previous chapters have placed on integrating patient education into their practices, consumer-prescribed information therapy may seem off-target. Why should we encourage people to search for information on their own? The answer comes in the three great advantages of consumer-prescribed information: timeliness, support, and focus. Consider these advantages from the consumer's point of view:

- **Timeliness:** I know me best, and I am the first on the scene for any illness or injury. I am the first to notice changes in my symptoms. I can best judge when I am ready to focus on a health decision or make an important behavior change. For all these reasons, consumer-prescribed information has a timeliness advantage over other forms of information therapy.

- **Support:** Information in itself has little value. Only when I am able to apply what I've learned to my behaviors, decisions, or beliefs does information hold real benefit. Information therapy that comes from my friends, family members, or support groups is likely to come with offers of support. That support is important to me.

- **Focus:** My physician has many, many patients to think about. I have only one. If my illness is serious, I can give it top priority. I can dedicate my full resources to searching for the right information. If I go to a condition-specific support group, my efforts are extended by others who share my focus. Because of the incredible availability of medical research on the Internet, I can find new medical knowledge that my physician may not have yet received. If used well and in cooperation with my doctor, this information can work to my advantage.

The Challenges of Consumer-Prescribed Therapy

Consumer-prescribed information comes with risks too. If the information is of poor quality, it can inappropriately undermine the physician's efforts. If the information is not appropriate for the patient's current moment in care, it can confuse and distract the patient from what's important. And if the information is not well integrated with the efforts of the medical team, it can disrupt the doctor-patient relationship.

To avoid or at least limit these risks, people using consumer-prescribed information must be able to find Prescription-Strength Information, focus on a specific moment in care, and introduce the information to their clinicians. This goes for family and friends of patients as well as the patients themselves. When a person becomes ill, it is only natural for family and friends to want to help. Often the best help they can provide, in addition to expressing love and support, is finding information that will guide the ill person through the treatment and behavior change decisions that lie ahead.

The role of this "health friend" can shift, depending on the changing needs of the person with the illness. Often, all that the sick person needs is warm support and good wishes. Even so, a health friend to confide in and to share feelings and plans for recovery with can be extremely comforting. However, when the illness is serious and complex or the patient is very sick, the role of the health friend may quickly change to that of medical advocate or a participant in the decision process. In all of these roles, the health friend faces the same Ix challenges as the patient: finding good information that relates specifically to the moment in care and presenting it to the clinical team.

Challenge 1: Finding Prescription-Strength Information

The most common form of information therapy occurs when individuals search the Internet for information about their own health problems or those of their family or friends. Many people simply go to their favorite search engine like Yahoo!® or Google™, type in their symptom or condition, and wait a few seconds for the response. Unless the spelling is off, these searches generally yield a good number of hits, even for the rarest of conditions. How many of those hits are good ones? And how can a person separate the good ones from the bad?

As discussed in Chapter 2, it is now thought that search engines may be hazardous to your health. The results of search engine searches have three basic problems: too many responses, little prioritization of responses, and the lack of quality control. (See pages 19 to 22 for a full explanation of these findings.)

For these reasons, consumers are advised to seek alternatives to general searches when looking for good health information.

- Ask a tech-savvy doctor. Doctors comfortable with the Internet may be able to suggest a good site. Most people would trust the information from a Web site their doctor told them about. However, physician-recommended Web sites, while usually reputable and evidence-based, may treat alternative medical approaches very conservatively or not at all. A good place to begin searching for information about complementary medicine is www.nccam.nih.gov, the Web site of the National Center for Complementary and Alternative Medicine at the National Institutes of Health.

- Ask a local hospital. Increasingly, hospitals are adding medical content to their Web sites. These sites usually include locally developed information as well as information from a nationally recognized content source. If the local hospital does not have such information, try going to the www.LaurusHealth.com Web site, which is run by VHA, Inc.

- Check out the government's recommendations, most of which can be found at www.healthfinder.gov.

- Consider going to the Web sites of well-respected medical centers, such as the Mayo Clinic's www.MayoClinic.com. Although a good name is not a guarantee that the information will include what you need, it is usually a good indicator that the information has been well reviewed by medical specialists.

LaurusHealth

www.laurushealth.com

LaurusHealth, of Irving, Texas, was developed by VHA, Inc., a national cooperative of more than 2,200 community-owned hospitals. It provides VHA members with quality health information for their Web sites to help them streamline their Internet strategies and meet the goal of community outreach. LaurusHealth's mission is to "provide consumers access to current, reliable health information, peer-reviewed and approved by leading physicians, nurses, pharmacists and hospitals, enabling consumers, patients and physicians to make informed health care decisions."

LaurusHealth offers its community Web site to VHA hospitals, physician practices, and other health care organization members. These groups can either link to the core site or create their own customized site using the same medical content. LaurusHealth also provides customer relationship management resources and tools for enhanced customer retention and satisfaction.

Ix Applications

Because LaurusHealth.com® is an open site, any physician can use it to deliver basic Ix applications. VHA also works in close collaboration with HEALTHvision, a privately held company formed through a collaboration of VHA and Eclipsys Corporation, to offer customized and locally branded Web-based Ix solutions to hospitals and hospital systems. Additional information is at www.healthvision.com and on page 159.

Q & A with Peter Plantes, MD, chief operations officer

Q: *Who uses LaurusHealth?*

A: By end of year 2001, LaurusHealth health information was contracted to over 350 VHA health care systems representing over 813 health care facilities in over 147 media markets. In 2001, over 5.1 million unique visits occurred to LaurusHealth, representing over 1.6 million unique users. While consumers and patients of all ages use LaurusHealth, key user groups include women of childbearing age and people age 50 and older.

Q: *LaurusHealth was one of the first sites to be accredited under the URAC Health Web Site Accreditation Program. In what ways does LaurusHealth.com protect its users to a greater extent than other Web sites?*

A: Registered users at LaurusHealth.com are assured that none of their information is shared with outside entities, such as marketers or insurance companies. The URAC accreditation fully demonstrates that the stringent security measures we take to protect user information are exemplary.

Challenge 2: Focusing on a Specific Moment in Care

Once in a good health Web site, the consumer still has the problem of finding the information needed for the current moment in care. If the diagnosis has yet to be confirmed, it may not make sense to go directly to treatment options. Focusing more on information about diagnostic tests and exams might be more helpful. Reading a Web site from front to back usually will not get people to the information they need in the time they have to find it.

A better approach is to write out specific questions and use the site's navigation and search options to answer them. (Web sites' sponsors can help by adding question-based navigation features to their sites.)

Challenge 3: Introducing the Information to the Clinical Team

Perhaps the greatest challenge of self-prescribed information is the difficulty of sharing it with clinicians. Even the most caring and e-aware physician cringes at the sight of a patient with an armload of Internet downloads. With a busy clinic schedule and the regular flow of medical journals and "must do" readings, the physician may have little time to review a patient's downloads. Consumers can help facilitate the information-sharing process by:

1. Limiting the amount of information they give their clinicians. More than one or two pages at a time can be too much for many busy clinicians. Keep it short, keep it specific, and keep it reliable.

2. Focusing on the most relevant information, and asking a specific question in reference to it.

3. Clearly presenting the source and credentials of the information and where the clinician can get the full report. The more respect a clinician has for the information, the more seriously he or she will respond to it.

4. Listening to their clinician's response and recording what is helpful. "Health friends"—family members or friends who accompany the person to the visit— can help by being a second pair of eyes and ears.

Jackson Williams
Self-Referral

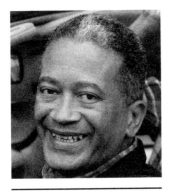

Search Results:

Coughs

☐ + Overview

☑ **+ Check Your Symptoms**

☐ + Home Treatment

☐ + Prevention

☐ + Preparing for Appt.

☐ + Related Information

☐ + Quitting Tobacco Use

Person: Jackson Williams

A few days after Jackson Williams saw Dr. Wood for his urinary problems (see page 52), he developed a "worse-than-usual" cough in that he was coughing up phlegm. Jackson is a pretty heavy smoker, and dry coughs are not unusual for him. He typically just "toughed it out" until the cough went away. This time, however, Jackson decided to look it up on the same Internet site that Dr. Wood had recommended for his urinary problem.

First he searched for "coughs" on the site and found three sections particularly helpful:

Coughs: Check Your Symptoms
Coughs: Home Treatment
Coughs: Prevention

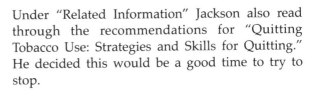

Under "Related Information" Jackson also read through the recommendations for "Quitting Tobacco Use: Strategies and Skills for Quitting." He decided this would be a good time to try to stop.

He found the information useful and decided to ask Dr. Wood about using a nicotine patch to help him quit.

Action Plan: Jackson developed the following plan:

1. Try home treatment: more liquids (up to 8 glasses of water a day) and an expectorant cough medication.

2. Stop smoking until the cough is gone (or cut back).

3. Try using nicotine patches to help quit smoking for good.

4. Call Dr. Wood to ask about over-the-counter versus prescription patches.

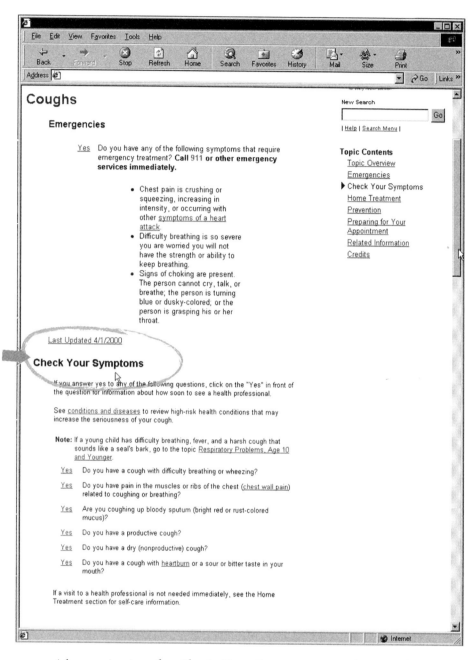

Coughs

Emergencies

Yes   Do you have any of the following symptoms that require emergency treatment? **Call 911 or other emergency services immediately.**

- Chest pain is crushing or squeezing, increasing in intensity, or occurring with other symptoms of a heart attack.
- Difficulty breathing is so severe you are worried you will not have the strength or ability to keep breathing.
- Signs of choking are present. The person cannot cry, talk, or breathe; the person is turning blue or dusky-colored; or the person is grasping his or her throat.

Last Updated 4/1/2000

Check Your Symptoms

If you answer yes to any of the following questions, click on the "Yes" in front of the question for information about how soon to see a health professional.

See conditions and diseases to review high-risk health conditions that may increase the seriousness of your cough.

Note: If a young child has difficulty breathing, fever, and a harsh cough that sounds like a seal's bark, go to the topic Respiratory Problems, Age 10 and Younger.

Yes   Do you have a cough with difficulty breathing or wheezing?

Yes   Do you have pain in the muscles or ribs of the chest (chest wall pain) related to coughing or breathing?

Yes   Are you coughing up bloody sputum (bright red or rust-colored mucus)?

Yes   Do you have a productive cough?

Yes   Do you have a dry (nonproductive) cough?

Yes   Do you have a cough with heartburn or a sour or bitter taste in your mouth?

If a visit to a health professional is not needed immediately, see the Home Treatment section for self-care information.

New Search

Go

| Help | Search Menu |

Topic Contents

Topic Overview

Emergencies

▶ Check Your Symptoms

Home Treatment

Prevention

Preparing for Your Appointment

Related Information

Credits

After reviewing the Check Your Symptoms questions, Jackson decided that an immediate clinic visit was not needed.

Lori Nelson

Referral by Family and Friends

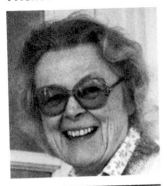

Search Results:

Osteoarthritis

- ☐ + Overview
- ☐ + Exams and Tests
- ☐ + Treatment Overview
- ☐ + Prevention
- ☐ + Home Treatment
- ☐ + Medications
- ☐ + Surgery
- ☑ + **Joint Replacement Surgery Decision**
- ☐ + Other Places to Get Help
- ☐ + Related Information

Patient: Lori Nelson

Family member: Mary Morrison

While Mary Morrison was clicking to information about her sinusitis (see page 49), she thought about her mother, 73-year-old Lori Nelson, and Lori's increasing trouble with her arthritic hips. Mary knew her mom was interested in the possibility of a hip replacement and had set an appointment for the following week to discuss it with her family physician.

After reviewing sections on "Hip Replacement Surgery" and "Making the Decision about Joint Replacement Surgery," Mary developed the following action plan to help her mom prepare for her appointment.

Action Plan: Mary developed the following plan:

1. Mary would send her mom the e-mail on page 123, which connects to decision-support information. This is a typical example of family- or friend-prescribed information therapy.

2. She would call her mom to ask if she had any questions about the information.

3. She would offer to go with her mom on the visit and to record what the doctor said.

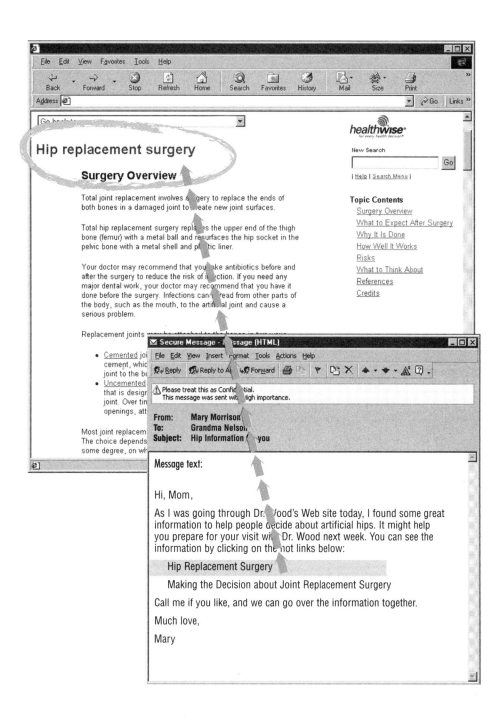

Support Group-Prescribed Information

Self-help and support groups help people cope with a broad spectrum of physical, mental, social, behavioral, and spiritual health issues. For many illnesses, patients in support groups value the information received from their peers. Support groups are particularly well developed and active in three areas:

- **Cancer.** There are hundreds of active support groups for people with cancer. Groups specialize in virtually every form of cancer from the most common to the rarest. These groups are not only helpful in understanding the risks and benefits of different treatment alternatives but can also guide people through the many nonmedical issues that cancer patients face.

- **Rare diseases.** Online support groups exist for almost every rare disease. For diseases that a physician may see only once in a lifetime of medical practice, it makes sense for patients to compare notes with other patients. Often these groups know far more about what works and doesn't work than many physicians do. At a minimum, they can refer others to physicians who specialize in the diagnosis and treatment of the disorder.

- **Diseases affecting children.** Parents often feel distressed and frustrated in dealing with their children's chronic illnesses and are grateful for the advice of others who have faced a similar situation. That common bond has created the needed ingredients for scores of active support groups of parents helping each other deal with their children's illnesses or disabilities.

Whatever the health problem, there is likely a support group somewhere that is focused just on it. The American Self-Help Clearinghouse maintains a periodically updated list of hundreds of self-help groups in the U.S. The list can be searched at www.mentalhelp.net/selfhelp.

It is important to recognize that not all self-help groups are created equal. The quality of the group depends largely on the level of volunteer effort put out by the leaders of the group. Some legitimate-looking groups can be "fronts" for companies or individuals wishing to promote and sell a particular product. However, such groups are in the small minority and can be avoided by shunning any groups that start promoting products of questionable merit.

Can support groups be purveyors of information therapy? To increase the value of their information in shared decision-making situations, self-help and support groups would do well to follow these guidelines in developing information packets for prescription to consumers:

• Organize information around moments in care to help consumers focus on their specific needs.

• Clearly separate opinion-based information from that which is evidence-based. Evidence-based information should be referenced to the literature.

• Include links to well-respected, medically reviewed, and accredited Web sites that confirm or supplement the group's information.

Billy Gomez

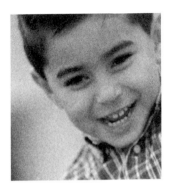

Patient: Billy Gomez
Family member: Alicia, his mom

Alicia Gomez has known for some time that her 6-year-old son, Billy, was "different" from other kids. Billy's kindergarten teacher told her she had seen a TV show about children who have a condition called Asperger's Syndrome, or AS.

Because the kids on the show reminded her of Billy, the teacher had written down the name of the Web site, www.aspergersyndrome.org, that the show mentioned.

When Alicia went to the Web site, she felt both relief and anxiety. As she read through the list of symptoms and the stories written by other parents, her thoughts amounted to, "This may be Billy." The Web site was run by parents of kids with AS, looked well-developed, and had won many Web quality awards. Alicia decided to send an e-mail to the site, asking for help in figuring out Billy's problem.

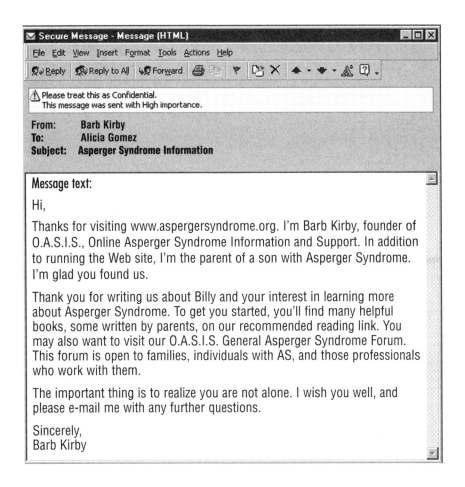

Secure Message - Message (HTML)

File Edit View Insert Format Tools Actions Help

Reply   Reply to All   Forward

⚠ Please treat this as Confidential.
    This message was sent with High importance.

From:	**Barb Kirby**
To:	**Alicia Gomez**
Subject:	**Asperger Syndrome Information**

Message text:

Hi,

Thanks for visiting www.aspergersyndrome.org. I'm Barb Kirby, founder of O.A.S.I.S., Online Asperger Syndrome Information and Support. In addition to running the Web site, I'm the parent of a son with Asperger Syndrome. I'm glad you found us.

Thank you for writing us about Billy and your interest in learning more about Asperger Syndrome. To get you started, you'll find many helpful books, some written by parents, on our recommended reading link. You may also want to visit our O.A.S.I.S. General Asperger Syndrome Forum. This forum is open to families, individuals with AS, and those professionals who work with them.

The important thing is to realize you are not alone. I wish you well, and please e-mail me with any further questions.

Sincerely,
Barb Kirby

O.A.S.I.S.: Online Asperger Syndrome Information and Support

www.aspergersyndrome.org

O.A.S.I.S. (Online Asperger Syndrome Information and Support) is typical of the many excellent support-group Web sites that have emerged on the Internet. O.A.S.I.S. is a Web site organized for and by parents of children who are diagnosed with Asperger Syndrome, or AS. It is also a vital meeting place for teens and adults with AS.

Asperger Syndrome (or Asperger's Disorder) is a neurobiological disorder named for a Viennese physician, Hans Asperger, who in 1944 published a paper that described a pattern of behaviors in several young boys who had normal intelligence and language development but who also exhibited autistic-like behaviors and marked deficiencies in social and communication skills. In spite of the publication of Asperger's paper in the 1940s, it wasn't until 1994 that Asperger Syndrome was added to the DSM-IV, and only in the past few years has AS been recognized by professionals and parents.

Written and maintained by a parent of a child with AS, O.A.S.I.S. maintains links with other organizations serving this community; reviews books and articles of interest to the AS community; and hosts forums for individuals with AS, parents, and health professionals.

"As parents of children who are diagnosed with AS, we understand how essential it is that families of children diagnosed with Asperger Syndrome and related disorders, educators who teach children with AS, professionals working with individuals diagnosed with AS, and individuals with AS who are seeking support, have access to information."

Barb Kirby, founder of O.A.S.I.S.

Population-Based Information Therapy: Moving Beyond the Individual

By definition, getting the right information to the right person at the right time focuses on the individual. However, population-based approaches that promote and support information therapy have been shown to be effective. Experimental community-based models that have exposed whole populations to mass information therapy have shown they can save money and save lives.

The community model of information therapy is based on three key elements: changing public expectations around self-care, self-management, and shared decision making; providing a common source of prescription-strength health information; and encouraging health professionals to prescribe information to their patients.

Changing Public Expectations

Not so very long ago, it was almost universal for people to think that "the doctor knows best" and that the patient should be "patient" and relatively passive. Over time, consumers' expectations have evolved slowly toward a model where patient and physician are partners. This shift in consciousness has occurred largely because of consumers' exposure to ever-increasing amounts of health and medical information and their belief that it is acceptable to play a more active role with their doctors.

More consumer involvement in health care is generally considered a good thing. There is growing evidence that self-care, self-management, and shared decision making are linked to improvements in outcomes and reductions in costs, both of which are sorely needed. Population-based programs can speed the public's adoption of consumer involvement in several ways. Foremost among them is the use of mass media to raise awareness about the acceptability of a more active role for consumers. In the following profiles of community-based models, you'll see how media ranging in sophistication from television ads to fliers sent to high school students were used to move public opinion toward an involved patient model. Publicly promoted workshops also allow people to both gain the new skills needed to practice self-care, self-management, and shared decision making and to discuss and process with others like themselves the changing role of the patient. Whether the workshops are happening in schools, senior centers, or church basements, recognition that others are trying on and having success with a more active role in health care encourages people to try it for themselves.

Providing a Common Source of Information

Population-based Ix approaches gain several advantages when they use a common source of Prescription-Strength Information across a community. If a community has access to a common source of information, clinicians can refer to it with an expectation that the patient will know about it and have access to it. And as clinicians become familiar with the content, they can more readily prescribe the right information to the right patient at the right moment in care. Making sure that no one is left out, population-based programs can also combine print, Internet, and a toll-free nurse care-counselor phone service to serve the information needs of everyone. And when everyone relies on the common source of information, the risk of providing contradictory or confusing information is greatly reduced.

Encouraging Clinicians to Prescribe and Support Information Therapy

Community-based programs have a better chance of gaining the attention and support of area clinicians than individual efforts. Many physicians may be unwilling to respond to the Ix efforts of a single managed care plan because doing so would impact only a fraction of their patients. Physicians are also notoriously busy coping with many demands upon their time and attention. A coordinated combination of mass media, targeted educational efforts, and "patient pull" can be required to gain the attention of a busy clinician. Community-based programs can use hospital grand rounds, medical society communications, and continuing medical education programs to raise clinician awareness and build new skills.

Physician expectations about the new consumer are important too. Learning new communication skills that can steer the patient's involvement in productive ways is far more satisfying than the frustration of dealing with "problem patients" when doctor-patient expectations don't match up. Combined with physicians' changing experiences with "new consumers," workshops approved as continuing medical education can help physicians lay down Ix strategies that will best serve the needs of their patients while enhancing the work flow and productivity of their practices.

Three Examples of Population-Based Programs

For the past 5 years, the community model described above has been in the demonstration and evaluation stage across North America. The profiles on pages 132 to 135 highlight efforts of varying size and scope in three different U.S. communities.

Bell County, Texas
www.phwise.org

Bell County sits in the rolling landscape of central Texas about midpoint between Austin and the Dallas-Fort Worth area. Boasting the cities of Killeen and Temple and a wide array of medical services, Bell County also hosts Hands on Health™, a collaborative, community-based, self-care program that is made available to employees of 29 Bell County employers and to the county's uninsured population. The Bell County Judge and Commissioners' Court administrates the funds: $400,000 raised from corporate donations, tobacco money, and county funds.

The vision for the Hands on Health program was to create a community of informed medical consumers in Texas. The goals of the program are to:

• Improve the practice of self-care for common health problems.

• Improve the appropriate use of medical services.

• Strengthen the partnership between patients and their health providers.

Hands on Health distributed a self-care book to the 16,000 employees of each of the participating Bell County employer groups and over 13,000 uninsured households. It also provides self-care workshops, seminars to help health care providers reinforce patients' use of the self-care book, and free access to a consumer information Web site.

A survey was sent to 100 uninsured households prior to program implementation. Respondents were asked, "Where do you go for health care?" Nine percent reported that they saw an MD, 23 percent said they went to a walk-in clinic, 66 percent reported going to the ER, and 2 percent said "other." Respondents were also asked how many times they went for medical services. Self-reported results after program implementation indicate that ER visits were reduced and that respondents were increasingly turning to health information services, particularly the self-care book and a telephone nurse, to answer their questions.

What has impressed project organizers most? The response of the uninsured population to having consumer health information resources. Michael Christ, who organized the education programs for the county's uninsured population, said, "People get it. Their eyes light up. No one wants to go sit and wait in an emergency room if they don't need to be there. It's making a definite difference with the uninsured of our county."

Partners Health Initiative
www.healthy-community.org

In the region around Anderson, South Carolina, the Partners Health Initiative (PHI), with support from 28 community sponsors, set out to create communities of informed health consumers in four local counties. They distributed free self-care handbooks to 146,000 households in 1999. They also set up the Partners Nursewise Line, a 24-hour nurse advice line. On its Web page, the project linked to a number of e-health sites that provide reliable consumer health information.

An independent evaluation was conducted using telephone surveys. Randomly selected households were polled before the initiative was launched and again at 6, 18, and 30 months. In addition, there was a medical utilization review for ambulatory care, hospitalization, and ER use, focusing on specific diagnostic codes.

Self-reported data gleaned from the telephone surveys at 18 months found:

- Use of the consumer information increased over time from 36 percent at 6 months to 40 percent.

- 23 percent reported avoiding an unnecessary visit to the doctor.

- 13 percent reported avoiding an unnecessary visit to the ER.

- An estimated $21 million was saved through reductions in unnecessary doctor and ER visits.

- The underinsured and uninsured were the greatest users of the consumer health information.

The PHI staff also surveyed the employees of sponsoring organizations after the first 6 to 8 months. Results indicated that 16 percent of this group saved at least one sick day.

The PHI team heard many stories of how consumers used the information available to them. One compelling story came from a young kindergarten teacher who experienced a severe headache while out on a bike ride. She stopped at a stranger's house and asked to use the phone to call her husband. While waiting for him to arrive, they looked through the program's self-care handbook and then called the Nursewise Line. The nurse told the woman in no uncertain terms to get to the emergency room, which she did. It turned out she was having a cerebral hemorrhage. She spent a week in the hospital but recovered fully. She credits the book and the Nursewise Line with saving her life.

Healthwise Communities Project, Idaho

www.healthwise.org/a_communities.html

In 1995, Healthwise, Incorporated, of Boise, Idaho, set out to help 280,000 Idahoans become the best-informed, most-empowered health care consumers in the world.

The Tools

- A *Healthwise® Handbook* in every home: Over 143,000 medical self-care guides were distributed to every household in a four-county area.

- The Healthwise® Knowledgebase: Every family had access to this electronic consumer health information database covering thousands of medical problems, drug therapies, and medical tests. Residents could access the Healthwise Knowledgebase via the "Healthwise Line," a telephone nurse advice line focusing on coaching, counseling, and shared decision making. During the study phase, more than 20,000 families—16 percent of the community—called for information. Healthwise "Information Stations," computer kiosks, were set up in over 50 libraries, clinics, and workplaces. At least 16,000 consumers used the kiosks to gather information about health and health care. There was also an open Web site that was used by an average 12,000 consumers every month.

- Consumer education: Workshops at schools, businesses, churches, and other venues taught skills in medical self-care and shared decision making.

- Provider education: In-service seminars taught 700 doctors, nurses, and other health professionals how to better work with informed medical consumers and how to use prescription information for better outcomes.

The Results

- **Consumers relied on the *Healthwise Handbook* as a trusted resource.** Medical self-care book use rose significantly—from 49 percent to 66 percent—and stayed up even 3 years after distribution of the book. Consumers used the book, on average, seven times per year. Of all book users:[1]

  - 84 percent reported their worry about a health problem was reduced.

  - 76 percent reported that they self-treated symptoms/health problems.

  - 56 percent reported that they saved a visit to a doctor.

  - 23 percent reported that they saved a visit to the ER.

- **Consumers reduced unnecessary medical visits.** The Idaho community noted a significant reduction for TLAS (time-limited acute symptom) visits.[2] There were 18.1 percent fewer visits to the ER.[3]

- **We saved money.** Consumers in the study area helped save between $7.5 million and $21.5 million by avoiding unnecessary ER and doctor office visits.

- **Doctors championed the Healthwise self-care initiative.**[4]

    - 91 percent of physicians said they wanted the *Healthwise Handbook* in their exam rooms.

    - 75 percent recommended the *Healthwise Handbook* to their patients.

    - 85 percent of physicians wanted their staff to have access to the Healthwise Knowledgebase.

    - 83 percent wanted their patients to use the Healthwise Knowledgebase.

- **Doctors made a difference.** Idahoans are more likely to report that a doctor encouraged them to use a medical self-care manual, and those encouraged were more likely to use one.[5]

In the end, the Healthwise Communities Project demonstrated that a population-wide educational program could change the self-care practices of an entire community and save millions of dollars.

Staff heard hundreds of success stories. A homeless man named Danny became the de facto consumer health information gatherer for other people living in a downtown Boise homeless shelter. He would collect their health questions, walk the four blocks to the Boise Public Library, do the research at the Healthwise Information Station there, and then report his findings back at the shelter.

We are confronted with insurmountable opportunities.

Pogo

7
Business Opportunities in Information Therapy

Information therapy opens up a world of business opportunities. The shift of the individual's role from "patient" to "partner" and the shift of information from being "about care" to being a "part of care" create new territories to be explored. How you weave value into your Ix offerings will make the difference between being a part of the leading edge or the bleeding edge.

A Cautionary Tale

Dot-bomb. Dot-compost. Dot-disaster. You've heard the catchphrases of the dot-com collapse. What was once heralded as The Next Big Thing in Health Care has taken a beating and is coming back only slowly. These early efforts did not fail because of a lack of capital. In the beginning, money flooded the e-health space at a staggering rate. Nor did most efforts fail because of inadequate technology. Many e-health initiatives were able to deliver the engineering side of their propositions. The dot-com ventures died because the solutions they offered didn't deliver a sustainable value proposition.

In order to achieve long-term success in today's health care arena, organizations need to deliver value. These areas stand out: managing costs, improving outcomes, and providing satisfaction.

The Value in Managing Costs

Health care is rife with perverse incentives. Because of contradictory reimbursement models—fee-for-service versus capitation—the potential value for the system does not always translate into real value for a particular part of the system. For example, a health plan that uses fully capitated contracts with physicians for primary care gets little short-term advantage from reducing the costs of primary care. And a physician paid on a fee-for-service basis has no incentive to reduce either the price per service or the frequency of services that lead toward high overall costs. To find success in the cost management model, the potential value must be aligned with incentives for the part of the system that is implementing the change.

Cost management comes in three basic forms: lowering the unit cost of a service; reducing the number of services delivered; and exchanging high-cost services with lower-cost services. Information therapy can add cost-management value in each of these three ways.

Lowering the Unit Cost of Patient Education

In clinics where high levels of patient education are already standard practice, the use of information prescriptions will save time and money. It is less costly and more effective to electronically push critical decision-support information than to rely solely on what the patient can remember from the clinic visit. It is also less costly to use electronic information than to manage stockpiles of printed handouts and brochures. The combination of less clinic time and better educational results would make for a good business proposition even if the effects of the education did not change any clinical decisions or prevent treatment mistakes. Because information therapy does lead to better outcomes, however, lowering the unit cost of education is only one of the ways information therapy can enhance value.

Reducing the Number of Medical Tests, Medications, and Procedures

Studies show that fully informing patients of the risks and benefits of treatment options improves patient outcomes and reduces costs. In essence, many patients are risk averse, and delivering the right information to the right person at the right time can lead to more conservative treatment decisions. An oft-cited research study involving a group of benign prostatic hyperplasia (BPH) patients found that fully informing patients of the side effects and outcome statistics associated with various treatment choices improved patient satisfaction and reduced surgery rates.[1] Other similar Ix applications that can be shown to result in fewer services without a loss in perceived quality or successful clinical outcomes will have strong value propositions for any organization that shares in the cost of care.

Of course, informed decision making will not yield immediate cost reductions in every medical situation, nor should it. In searching for quality medical care, we would hope to see an increase in utilization for underutilized but valuable services. Take, for example, disease management for people with diabetes. Routine screening of kidneys, feet, and eyes and preventive laser eye treatments improve long-term outcomes but are more costly. The strength of the evidence justifies these procedures, despite the cost. Correctly delivered, Ix prescriptions would likely increase the utilization rate and the related costs, at least in the short term. This short-term increase needs to be balanced against the potential improvements in patient outcomes and the long-term cost of care.

Exchanging High-Cost Services With Lower-Cost Services

In medicine the best care is often not the most expensive care. Information therapy, informing patients of their choices, can help make a high-cost item a lower-cost item. At the mundane, everyday end of the scale, for instance, self-care for a time-limited upper respiratory infection (get rest, drink liquids, take aspirin) is more cost-effective than professional care (a doctor telling the patient to get rest, drink liquids, and take aspirin) and produces the same clinical outcome. At the high end of the cost scale, some treatments previously available only through hospitalization are now available on an outpatient basis. For example, traditionally, a patient with deep vein thrombosis is admitted into hospital care for a 3- to 5-day stint of anticoagulation treatment.

Studies now show that an alternative treatment is available that allows the patient to stay at home and receive equally effective and safe treatment.[2] True, the actual medication used in the home program is more expensive than the hospital-based medication, but the patient avoids the costs and risks of hospitalization.

When educated and informed about their options, such as this one, patients may show the same tendency toward conservative treatment options that they show for surgical decisions. Information therapy applications that can help patients and their physicians discover the most appropriate treatment to achieve their goals—positive outcomes—can create and demonstrate value.

The Value in Improving Outcomes

The underlying value of health care comes from helping sick people become well and well people stay healthy. The basic premise of this book is all about how getting the right information to the right person at the right time improves outcomes. Ix applications that can demonstrate significant improvements in outcomes throughout the health care continuum have the basics for a strong value proposition.

The Value in Providing Satisfaction

When satisfaction levels go up, patient loyalty to both physicians and health plans improves as well. The resulting improvement in market share and turnover rates can make a difference in the financial viability of a clinic or plan. Information therapy can add another important factor to improving and ensuring both patient and provider satisfaction.

Every clinical encounter affects patient-clinician satisfaction, for good or ill. Clinician-prescribed information prescriptions reinforce the positive. Via these prescriptions, doctors help patients understand their conditions, their treatment plans, and their self-management options. They also say, "I care about you." And they help meet the doctor's need to provide the best in quality health care.

Information prescriptions also provide an opportunity for health plans to communicate with their members on issues other than claims and costs and premiums. Informational contacts from the plan to the patient that focus on quality decisions, not cost, add a positive dimension to the relationship.

Other Considerations

Managing costs, improving outcomes, and providing satisfaction could be considered the "golden goals" for any health care organization. If you're making good headway on all three of these fronts, your organization is probably more viable than most. Here are two additional considerations: make your Ix offerings truly consumer-centric, and keep them as simple as can be.

Consumer-Centric: The "Do-It-With-Me" Consideration

Many business thinkers in health care have paid little attention to the term "patient-centered." Helping doctors and nurses better focus on each patient may seem akin to motherhood and apple pie—a nice idea, but where's the profit in it? The profit lies in giving consumers what they are looking for.

Ignoring the consumer or patient-centric concept is no longer an option. Consider current trends in e-banking, e-finance, e-travel, and even e-news. It is all "me"-centric. The Internet allows the world to be interpreted and presented as each person wants it. Don't think that health care will be an exception. Any e-health solution that fails to place or support the patient at the center of care will be passed over as the new standard of patient-centered care gains dominance. While the patient-centered movement may not yet have won over all of health care, it has won over the segment of the population most attracted to e-health. These health information seekers are at the vanguard of the new paradigm and will accept nothing less than a patient-centered future.

For Ix applications, there are a few lessons to be learned:

- **It's got to be participatory**. For most of us, patienthood used to be a fairly passive experience. If our doctor gave us a medication prescription, we would just take it. The compliance model was king. If information therapy follows the same passive route of "receive and comply," chances are it will be of little interest to the new consumer. Only when the information is used to encourage participation in medical decisions or care management will it strike the needed consumer-centric note. The prescription should be a starting point that opens the door for consumers to gain access to good information that is directly related to their problem. Whether they go through the door and how far they explore is up to them.

- **The information has to be open**. Prescription-Strength Information can give the impression that some information is available only by prescription. Any e-health application that follows that assumption is doomed to failure. In general, no information should be off-limits to the patient. Just as full access to medical records has been established as a patient's right, full access to evidence-based medical knowledge should be considered a given.

- **It must be supportive of consumer choice**. In this new era of medicine, informed patient autonomy is the standard. The clinician's role is to inform and advise but not to overrule reasonable decisions by the patient. In the patient-centered world, the rule is clear: "Nothing about me, without me."

Information therapy and other e-health solutions that encourage consumer participation, that give open access to information, and that are actively supportive of shared decision making have a far better chance of success than those that do not.

Practical: The "Keep-It-Simple" Consideration

To be effective, information therapy has to be easy and intuitive for both the clinician and the patient. Don't get too fancy. Information therapy solutions that are complex or confusing or that require too many extra steps in the work flow of a busy practice will fail. Even if the value proposition is strong and the patient values the service, the application will never make it out of the pilot project stage if it is a hassle for clinicians or system administrators to implement.

Decision tools that require clinicians to go through detailed and time-consuming explanations of alternatives treatments are not built for success. There just isn't time for "standard gamble," "time trade-off," or other in-depth decision analysis techniques in a busy practice. Anything that takes much more than an extra minute of clinic time is a nonstarter. Even an extra minute raises suspicion. The applications that succeed will take place either outside of clinic time or in a way that reduces the net clinic time.

Fortunately, information therapy can be delivered with simplicity. Although the algorithms for selecting the right information for the right person at the right time can be complex, all of the complexity lives inside the computer. To the clinician clicking to send an information prescription or to the patient receiving it, the mechanics of information therapy can and should be simplicity itself.

Connecting Business Opportunities to Information Therapy

We live in a complex world. Health care used to be what happened between a patient and a doctor, and occasionally the hospital. Now, it's what happens between a patient and a doctor and the health insurer and the clinic and the hospital and the Internet and the disease management company, ad infinitum. In this section we highlight ten health care business environments and look at the value propositions and opportunities for information therapy in each one.

Remember the seven opportunities for information therapy as described on pages 41 to 43: prevention, self-care, self-triage, visit preparation, self-management of chronic disease, decision support, and end-of-life care. In the e-health world, virtually every one of them is open to every e-health business plan. Table 7.1 on page 144 ranks the significance of the opportunity. (The more dots, the more significant the opportunity.)

Table 7.1 E-Health Value-Opportunity Matrix

E-health Business Plan Focus	Prevention	Self-care	Self-triage	Visit prep	Self-mgt. of chronic disease	Decision support	End-of-life care
Health Plans	••	•••	•••	•	•••	•••	•••
Consumer-Driven Plans	••	•••	••	•	•••	•••	•••
Hospitals	•	•••	•	•••	•••	•••	•••
Clinics	•••	••	•••	•••	••	••	••
Physician-to-Patient Portals	•••	•••	•••	•••	•••	•••	•••
Electronic Medical Records	•••	•	•		•••	•••	•••
Transaction Companies	•	•	•	•	•••	•••	•••
Decision-Support Services	••	•••	•••	•••	••	•••	•••
Pharmacy Benefit Management					••	••	
Disease Management	•	•••	••	•	•••	•••	•••

Note: The more dots, the more significant the opportunity.

Managed Care Organizations

For traditional managed care organizations (MCOs), business success is based on a plan's ability to manage high-quality care more effectively than its competitors. The business measures most important to an MCO include membership (size, growth, and retention); the medical benefit ratio (the percent of premium that goes to pay claims or provide medical services); and the administrative cost ratio (the percent of premium needed for administration of the plan). If the membership is growing (and membership "churn" or turnover is minimized), and if the two ratios combined leave a substantial and consistent profit, the plan is successful.

To maximize results for these three measures, MCOs must engage in a complex array of activities aimed not just at its members but also at the physicians and hospitals who give them care and at the employers who pay their premiums. Information therapy applications can help an MCO attain its goals in all three of its key measures.

Membership

Membership growth is based on premium, coverage, and service competitiveness. To an MCO, growing membership is important only if the combination of premium rate and cost of care result in a profit. Of particular importance is the need to reduce churn, or turnover of members. Losing old members while gaining new members at every open enrollment costs administrative dollars. Whether its plan is to attract or keep members, a plan must be "a good deal" in the minds of both the consumer and the employer who is purchasing the benefit. Information therapy, as a benefit of enrollment, can positively impact the rate of churn because it helps make the plan seem like a good deal.

Selection bias also needs to be considered. Whenever a plan offers a new benefit, it considers the kind of new member that will be attracted to the offering. Will the new benefit appeal to high utilizers or low utilizers of care? Given the demographics of health information seekers, information therapy creates a positive selection bias. Educated, motivated, and involved patients are more likely to use services appropriately.

Medical Benefit Ratio

In medical care, more is not always better. A sizeable portion of currently provided medical services provides little or no benefit to the patient, but denial of these services, either through claims denial or utilization review, pleases no one. Patients get angry and physicians are put at odds with the plan. This all-around negative situation undermines the value proposition of the plan. MCOs and physicians could alleviate this situation by providing information prescriptions of evidence-based information at the time of a major decision. Information therapy helps consumers to better understand their options and educates them more fully on the pros and cons of any particular treatment. Rather than being denied a service because it's not appropriate, a well-informed patient will be less likely to request the service in the first place. An MCO or a physician is much more likely to get patient buy-in if the patient is given all the facts and allowed to participate in the decision.

Administrative Cost Ratio

Information therapy applications can reduce administrative costs in two ways. First, costs associated with delivering and monitoring patient education for National Committee for Quality Assurance (NCQA) accreditation standards and medical and legal purposes can be reduced through Ix technology. Second, though admittedly more long-term, as information prescriptions become reimbursable, the cost of providing them shifts into the medical services category (information as therapy), hence reducing the administrative cost ratio.

Different Strokes for Different MCOs

Group model health maintenance organizations (HMOs) like Kaiser Permanente and Group Health Cooperative have the capability to act on all seven of the Ix opportunities for health care improvement. However, the opportunities open to other health plans may differ greatly, depending on the comprehensiveness and integration of their health information systems. Real-time access to preauthorization requests, claims data, test data, and medication data is needed to trigger information prescriptions. The more an MCO's data warehouse has current, accurate, and integrated information, the better able the plan is to deliver effective information prescriptions.

Kaiser Permanente
www.kp.org

Kaiser Permanente (KP) is America's largest not-for-profit health maintenance organization. It began as a health plan in the 1930s for the Kaiser industries' construction, shipyard, and mill workers. The plans were open to community enrollment in 1945 and have since grown to cover over 8 million people in nine states and the District of Columbia.

Today, Kaiser Permanente encompasses Kaiser Foundation Health Plan, Inc., Kaiser Foundation Hospitals, and the Permanente Medical Groups as well as affiliation with Group Health Cooperative based in Seattle, Washington. Kaiser Permanente aspires to be the world leader in improving health through high-quality, affordable, integrated health care. KP's mission is "to provide affordable, quality health care services and to improve the health of our members and the communities we serve."

Kaiser has long been a center of excellence in health education. Health education is integrated into its clinical services, and Kaiser health educators have provided national leadership in expanding both the art and the science of health education. Kaiser has pioneered the development of health education centers as well as primary care teams and chronic conditions management programs in which physicians, nurses, pharmacists, nutritionists, health educators, and other professionals share the responsibilities of care. Finally, by encouraging member self-care and shared decision making, Kaiser has welcomed its members to join its primary care teams.

Ix Applications

Kaiser has supported consumer-prescribed information therapy for years. By giving each member a self-care handbook and encouraging its use through member communications and clinician referrals, Kaiser has created a culture in which members often look up and care for their own health problems upon the first signs of a new symptom. The addition of KP Online in recent years has enabled Kaiser members to find in-depth information on virtually any health problem without leaving the Kaiser Web site. By adding appointment scheduling, prescription drug refills, lab test reporting to members, and other clinical support services, KP Online is now well-positioned to begin pushing the same in-depth information to members at the right time to help them make better health decisions.

147

Group Health Cooperative
www.ghc.org

Group Health Cooperative (GHC) is a Seattle-based, consumer-governed, not-for-profit health care system that integrates health care and coverage. The Group Health system includes 2 hospitals, 28 primary care centers, 5 specialty centers, and close to 10,000 staff, including over 1,000 physicians. It serves nearly 600,000 members in Washington and northern Idaho. GHC is governed by a Board of Trustees elected by Group Health members. Member participation in the governance has led to a strong emphasis on member education and involvement in medical decisions.

In August 2000, MyGroupHealth, an Internet portal for patients with secure, Web-based messaging between patients and their health care teams, was completed across 23 medical centers.

Ix Applications

Group Health has outlined a four-phase, multiyear program to help patients perform self-management, and shared decision making using MyGroupHealth.

- Phase I includes physician-prescribed information delivered in clinics.

- Phase II includes health care team-prescribed information delivered in the medical centers, plus secure messaging.

- Phase III includes system-prescribed information delivered online.

- Phase IV includes automated, system-prescribed information delivered in the context of a patient-viewable personal health record.

All of this sits on top of a long-standing member health Web site that offers in-depth, searchable health content on most medical problems.

In Phase I, Group Health helps its clinicians write information prescriptions by publishing a "Hotlist" that links high-frequency diagnosis codes with medical content. By looking up the health problem by diagnosis code or problem name, the clinician can quickly find a predetermined link to guide the patient to relevant information. The clinician then writes a prescription for the information that the patient can search for on MyGroupHealth or that can be printed for the patient in the medical center. Phase II extends the service to member requests for information that arrive via secure messages to the health care team.

First Health
www.firsthealth.com

First Health® is a national health benefits company, providing large, multi-sited employers with an integrated solution for all their group health benefits needs. First Health was founded in 1982 as a utilization review company named HealthCare COMPARE Corp. The company changed its name in 1998 to better communicate the depth and range of its services. Today, the company offers two separate national preferred provider organizations (PPOs), pharmacy benefit management services, claims administration, stop-loss insurance, as well as clinical management services.

Ix Applications

First Health combines in its 24/365 call center a personal response service for consumer questions about coverage, eligibility, claim status, provider locations, and general health information. The same information is also available to consumers through the My First Health® Web site. Through My First Health® and their own secure sites, consumers can explore details about their benefit plans, check medical claims status for each covered member of the family, or locate doctors and hospitals that participate in The First Health® Network. With the online general health information database, they can access comprehensive, up-to-date health information any time they need it.

In addition, First Health is developing new programs that facilitate the Web-based interaction between plan members and network physicians. First Health's Internet Visit pilot program is testing the feasibility of paying physicians for virtual visits that consist of an e-mail and response for problems that might otherwise have required an in-person visit. Each such "Internet visit"—an e-mail and response, or more than one exchange on one topic—will pay the doctor $25. Patients who are part of the First Health Care Support program will be entitled to up to two "visits" a month. Company officials predict that the Internet visits will more than pay for themselves if they help chronically ill patients avoid acute episodes that often result in costly hospital stays.

Consumer-Directed Health Plans

Some say the current American health care financing system of employer-brokered health insurance is an idea whose time has passed. This long-established and paternalistic system was originally based on four primary assumptions, namely, there's a single wage earner in a nuclear family; there's lifetime employment with the same employer; one size of insurance fits all; and consumers are uninformed about their health care options. These assumptions are no longer valid.

By jettisoning these assumptions and focusing on the new realities of twenty-first-century health care, a new industry has emerged: consumer-directed health care. (Because many of these plans also allow for the employer to place a limit on its financial risks, some of these plans are also known as defined contribution plans. However, the term "consumer-directed" is much more representative of their core nature.)

Consumer-directed health plans operate under different assumptions than traditional employer-brokered health plans. They assume that consumers are looking for greater control, more choices, and a stronger doctor-patient relationship. They also assume that physicians and other providers are eager to exercise more freedom in the way that they practice medicine and care for patients. In short, consumer-directed plans propose that patients and doctors can fulfill health care needs more effectively than a managed care organization or an insurance company.

In a consumer-directed plan, an employer deposits funds into an employee's personal account. This money is then used to pay for the employee's health needs. The telling difference is that each employee chooses how to spend his or her health benefit dollars. There are no restrictions on which doctor an employee can see and what kind of treatments an employee can have. Any funds remaining in the account at the end of the year then roll over and stay with the employee. (Plans also arrange for supplemental coverage for unexpected or major health care costs.)

Proponents of consumer-directed plans argue that better-informed employee/patients can improve outcomes and lower costs. In order to help keep employees informed, these plans make available a host of health information and care management tools to help consumers navigate the health care system and to make better health care decisions.

Consumer-directed health plans use differing approaches and business plans to give individuals more choice in how their employer-sponsored health dollars are directed. Each is exploring its own solutions to the critical issues of risk adjustment and adverse selection so critical to long-term success. But common among all these plans is the use of technology and education to give people more control over their health care purchases. Again, the assumption is that giving consumers more ownership of and information about their care will lead to more responsible decisions and better overall value for the resources spent.

Because education is a core strategy among all consumer-driven plans, information therapy will play a strong role in determining the industry's success. If using the right information at the right time helps people make better decisions, this new form of health care financing will be a great success. If not, high costs and poor outcomes will endanger the viability of this new model.

In March 2001, eight plans came together to form the Consumer Driven Health Care Association (www.cdhca.org). The founding members included Definity Health, Destiny Health, HealthAllies, HealthMarket, Lumenos, Myhealthbank, Sageo, and Vivius. Each is described briefly below. (Please note that consolidations and market success may quickly change the landscape for this emerging industry.)

- **Definity Health** (www.definityhealth.com)

Minneapolis-based Definity Health offers a three-part product that gives consumers greater control over their own health care decisions and expenses. Each year the enrollee's employer deposits a fixed amount into a "Personal Care Account." The enrollee uses this account to pay for such things as eyeglasses, acupuncture, and chiropractic or dental services, in addition to traditional medical services. Choice of doctor and choice of service is decided by the enrollee. Any funds remaining at the end of the year are rolled over for the next year. Definity Health offers high-deductible coverage that is not used until the funds in the personal care account are depleted. They also employ information and care-management tools to help the consumer make better health and wellness decisions.

- **Destiny Health** (www.destinyhealth.com)

Destiny Health, based in Bethesda, Maryland, is a subsidiary of a South African company, Discovery Holdings, Ltd., which has enrolled close to a million members in consumer-driven health plans internationally. Enrollees of Destiny Health are provided a Personal Medical Fund™ from which they can withdraw funds to pay health care expenses. An additional comprehensive insurance benefit covers hospital and surgical needs, chronic disease medication needs, and "safety net" coverage if day-to-day expenses exceed an annual threshold.

- **HealthAllies** (www.healthallies.com)

HealthAllies in Glendale, California, provides a system for discounted consumer purchasing of health care services through contracts arranged through their employers. HealthAllies' approach is to provide a "time-of-need network" to supplement existing health insurance products. While HealthAllies does not replace the insurance function, they do allow for a managed system of care for such things as laser eye surgery, orthodontics, cosmetic dentistry, family counseling, travel immunizations, acupuncture, massage therapy, and prescription drugs.

- **HealthMarket** (www.healthmarket.com)

Founded in 1999 in Norwalk, Connecticut, HealthMarket offers consumers a HealthMarket Savings Account. The account is funded by the employer and provides first-dollar coverage for routine and preventive care, such as annual checkups, mammograms, allergy testing, and a variety of other preventive measures. HealthMarket's Self Directed Health Plan concept includes direct-to-consumer information services that compare the price and quality of different health care providers before seeking services. The company's Web site and telephone services also have extensive consumer health information to foster more informed decision making.

- **Lumenos** (www.lumenos.com)

Based in Alexandria, Virginia, Lumenos is a consumer-driven health plan that provides a Lumenos Health Savings Account plus a Health Toolkit to help members manage their health decisions wisely. The Toolkit both provides health information and helps track medical expenses. Lumenos has also negotiated discounts with many service providers for its members. There is also a comprehensive insurance plan that kicks in after the Health Savings Account is depleted. Year-to-year rollovers of unspent amounts in the account allow the buildup of savings for significant medical events in the future.

- **MyHealthBank** (www.myhealthbank.com)

Portland, Oregon-based MyHealthBank provides employers with an Internet-based health benefit service designed to give employees greater control over their health benefits and health care. Using MyHealthBank's platform, employers define their financial contribution for their group's underwritten employee health benefits. Employees select from a menu of insurance coverage options the level of coverage they want, allowing them to pay or retain the difference between their employers' contribution and the cost of their coverage.

- **Sageo** (www.sageo.com)

Founded by management consulting firm Hewitt Associates, Sageo provides a service through employers that helps the consumer select and use the health plan and benefits that are best suited to them. The Lincolnshire, Illinois-based firm offers a selection of hundreds of health plans from across the country to participating employers. Sageo's customer care service and Internet-based information system provide members with a wide range of information to help them understand their health care needs and select care providers.

- **Vivius** (www.vivius.com)

Based in Minneapolis, Vivius offers a health care purchasing account, a personalized panel of providers and a comprehensive insurance program. The Vivius plan allows consumers to select their own panel of clinicians and the level of co-pay that they want to use with each. A "wrap" plan covers the services provided outside of the main plan.

For these new companies and their consumer-driven focus to succeed, they will need to address the principles of value, consumer-centricity, and practicality discussed earlier in this chapter. The consumer-centric principle is well established. Value enhancement is certainly possible via cost reduction. The plans give the consumer a financial incentive to make cost-effective decisions that should lead to reductions in unnecessary care. Even greater savings may come by eliminating much of the high cost associated with claims processing, approval, denial, and payment. Additional savings will come from Web-based solutions to the selection and management of each employee's health plan relationship. Consumer-directed plans also anticipate a favorable selection bias since, historically, their approach attracts low utilizers of health care services: younger individuals and families who want to exercise more control over their health care options. (Note: The potential for savings looks good, but at this early stage in the industry, there has been little evidence of proof.)

In the end, the practicality principle may be the one most critical for consumer-directed health plans. If managing a medical savings account proves to be tedious, confusing, or prone to errors, the fate of consumer-driven health plans may be a fast rise and fall in the marketplace. On the other hand, if these plans use innovative technology to simplify payment and reimbursement, that simplicity alone could secure their long-term positive future.

Hospitals

Hospitals have significant incentives and opportunities for using information therapy to enhance both their missions and their bottom lines. They are also faced with major challenges.

Hospitals, whether nonprofit or investor-owned, are all businesses. Most are big businesses with thousands of employees and hundreds of diagnostic, therapeutic, and support services. In the midst of a mind-boggling collection of externally imposed regulations, hospitals must accurately bill for and collect millions of dollars just to keep their doors open.

In competitive markets, hospitals are challenged to attract both patients and good staff to their facilities and their ancillary medical services. (And increasingly, all markets are competitive.) To attract patients, hospitals need to put some muscle behind their promises to be patient-centered. They need to meet patient demand for more treatment information and involvement in treatment decisions.

Hospital leaders have been challenged by the reports of preventable medical mistakes and systems errors that erode patient safety and, at times, lead to death or significant harm for the patients under their care. The industry leaders on the boards of community hospitals have become increasingly intolerant of the high-cost and poor-quality performance that they see. Leading hospital systems are now positioning themselves to provide a patient-safety, patient-centered response that for the first time seems strong enough to make a difference.

Hospitals cannot serve patients without first attracting physicians to practice in their facilities. To attract and keep physicians, hospitals compete based on convenience; access to the tests, equipment, and procedures that are the standard of care for the community; competent support; and a foundation of quality. A hospital's support of top-quality information therapy can become one more inducement.

Hospitals also need to be nurse-focused to survive. At this writing, American health care is facing a critical shortage of nurses and a remarkable level of discontent among nurses in practice. According to a survey conducted by the American Nurses Association, "an overwhelming number of nurses have experienced an increased patient load for RNs resulting in a dramatic decrease in the quality of care." A majority of nurses responding to the survey believe that their time available for direct patient care has decreased: "Care has declined because of inadequate staffing, decreased nurse satisfaction and a delay in providing basic care."[3] From the nurses' point of view, things are not good.

Can technology be employed to meet the needs of patients and clinicians? Many hospital systems have already made multimillion-dollar investments in information technology. For those who have made the investment in these technologies, every department is computerized, every service is electronically tracked, and every bill is digital. Most hospital Web sites now deliver both marketing information about the hospital's services and searchable health information for their communities. Their greatest Ix opportunities now come in piggybacking information prescriptions on top of technological advances in ways that satisfy both patients and clinicians, while raising hospital revenues, reducing costs, or reducing preventable mistakes. Four piggyback approaches appear most attractive: robust information prescriptions as a part of call center information services; wireless device-aided information prescriptions; system-prescribed information therapy; and digital bedsides.

Call Center Services

Information therapy has a big role in the call center, turning it from a triage and physician referral "shop" into a significant initiative to improve the quality of care. Information therapy, delivered via a hospital-based, nurse-staffed call center, also gives nurses the tools to fulfill one of their primary professional functions—the education of the patient.

Wireless Device-Aided Information Prescriptions

Many hospitals have begun implementing wireless systems that allow computer-aided order entry for physicians and other professionals in the course of clinical care. The value proposition being pursued is based on a combination of convenience and quality enhancement. If the clinician can order drugs, tests, or procedures right on the spot with the patient, it can mean less paperwork, fewer errors due to misinterpreted handwriting, and fewer orders that are inadvertently outside of quality standards. Once a clinician learns and embraces such a system, it theoretically becomes a strong attraction for using the hospital and the hospital's services.

Hospitals implementing wireless systems can gain further advantage by tapping their potential for information prescriptions. With no more than a click or two on the handheld device, a clinician can add an information prescription to every order entry done through a wireless system. In many cases the information prescriptions can be done automatically with no additional clicks at all.

The hospital value proposition for wireless-enhanced information prescriptions is threefold:

1. **Work flow efficiency**. Wireless prescriptions allow physicians, nurses, and other clinicians to educate their patients and document informed consent more effectively and in less time than current practice. In some cases the impact of the improvements will be dramatic and will result in earlier discharge and fewer hospital readmissions.

2. **Patient satisfaction**. Information therapy builds satisfaction and loyalty among those patients who want more information and involvement in their care. Satisfied patients will result in increased market share and donor support.

3. **Clinical quality**. Information prescriptions add a final, patient-centered quality check on all clinical services that can prevent medical errors and assure that the likely treatment outcomes are aligned with the patient's preferences and expectations.

For certain patients, order-entry information prescriptions to the patient and family can help their efforts effectively add to the professional care provided. Eventually, such self-help efforts may lessen the burden of understaffing plaguing hospitals today.

System-Prescribed Information Therapy

Hospital information systems are usually made up of numerous, separately developed special-purpose subsystems that serve the many departments and functional areas of the hospital. Labs, billing, and patient care all tend to speak a separate language. When it comes to information technology systems, a hospital can resemble an electronic Tower of Babel. Help is on the way, though, to ease the translation from one system to another. Interface standards such as HL7 (Health Level 7) help diverse systems communicate in a common format, if not a common language. Also, new standards are currently being developed that focus on the "clinical context" of information objects across all applications. For instance, a change made to a patient's ER chart about a medication allergy would be picked up systemwide so that separate and duplicated entries aren't needed and records are kept up to date. Piggyback applications using CCOW (Clinical Context Object Workgroup) will increasingly allow information from many different subsystems to be used in triggering the right information for the right patient at the right time. Systems integration will aid in achieving more precise information prescriptions, adding to all of the benefits described above for wireless applications. (There's more discussion about HL7, CCOW, and the language of triggers on pages 103 to 107.)

Digital Bedsides

Forward-thinking hospitals envision patient bedside computers being as ubiquitous and commonplace as today's bedside telephones. Innovative hospitals have begun to experiment with devices like tablet PCs and Webpads that provide wireless online connections. Currently employed to link patients with e-mail and popular Web sites, wireless access to Ix applications will bring to bedside computers a much higher level of value and truly integrate the patient and the family into the care team. With all medical orders, lab results, medical history, and other important information available for 24/7 review, patients and their families will be able to prepare for each next step in treatment and to help prevent medical errors or catch them early, if they occur.

The value proposition for hospitals that adopt this approach early is positive public relations and patient satisfaction combined with the benefits and cost savings that come from lower medical error rates and greater work flow efficiency.

Getting Launched

Hospitals don't need to wait for high-tech, piggyback opportunities to get started with information therapy. In some hospital departments, the need for and the value of information prescriptions are so great that paper-based checklists make sense for immediate use. All that is needed is Prescription-Strength Information on a patient-accessible Web site and a way for clinicians to give each patient the specific URL to the precise information they need.

HEALTHvision
www.healthvision.com

HEALTHvision™ is focused on providing local hospitals, clinics, and other health care delivery organizations with Internet-based solutions that connect physicians, patients, consumers, and employees. HEALTHvision provides its clients with an integrated framework for a broad range of Internet-enabled services that can be presented under the branding of the local organization.

HEALTHvision was formed in 1999 as a joint venture between VHA and Eclipsys. VHA is a Texas-based health care alliance with over 1,800 health care organization members. Eclipsys is a provider of outcomes-focused health care information technology solutions.

Ix Applications

HEALTHvision offers two primary products with information therapy implications: COMMUNITYvision and CAREvision.

COMMUNITYvision provides each client with a consumer health portal that establishes the client's reputation as a trusted source of information in the community. The COMMUNITYvision portals provide the source information for a great variety of consumer-prescribed Ix applications, as discussed in Chapter 6. In addition to health content, COMMUNITYvision provides opportunities for local organizational news, physician directories, education workshop schedules, and other information to be posted on the portal. The look and feel of the portal is customizable to support the branding and core messages of the local organization.

CAREvision provides participating organizations with a secure messaging system to send information to their patients, as well as Internet-based prescription management, order entry, care management, and clinical referral capabilities. In addition, CAREvision provides the capabilities to automatically send patients lab results, to provide clinicians current clinical content, and to provide free text support for medical notes.

Each CAREvision application provides a rich source of information triggers for the future deployment of information prescriptions to patients. HEALTHvision has invested heavily in content improvements that will allow prescription information to be targeted to the specific decision or moment in care a particular patient is facing.

Clarian Health

www.clarian.org

Clarian Health is an Indiana-based private, not-for-profit organization comprised of Methodist Hospital, Indiana University Hospital, and Riley Hospital for Children. Collectively known as Clarian Health, the organization's mission is to improve the health of patients and the community through innovation and excellence in care, education, research, and service.

Ix Applications

Clarian's Web site was developed to provide patients with personalized Web site content that includes:

• The ability to create a highly secure "MyClarian" account in which members can store favorite articles and their physicians' information.

• Health tips targeted to a patient's health interests.

• Downloadable palm pilot applications for patients to track their personal health.

• Physician-reviewed health care content.

• The Find-a-Doctor tool and online appointment scheduling.

• Secured online requests for personal medical records and itemized bill request.

• Secure online hospital bill payment.

• A site for referring physicians.

Q & A with Tal Moise, vice president of Business Innovations

Q: *What's planned for the future?*

A: We will continue to make many enhancements, such as the ability to create and store personal medical records, as well as an option to have an emergency medical card created with that data. Information therapy will be an advanced personalization tool on Clarian's Web site that will allow consumers to receive personalized health information and preventive care advice.

Clarian is developing a system to compile dynamic profiles of registered visitors and, through clinical rules, determine what health information would be appropriate for a given person. The end result will be a continually changing profile with personalized information directed to the user. Individuals will have the opportunity to opt in or out of having their profiles developed.

Our goal is to bring high-quality health care information to consumers via their Web sites and remain in touch with patients before and after they visit one of Clarian's facilities.

Memorial Hospital and Health System
www.qualityoflife.org

Memorial Hospital and Health System is a private, independent, community-owned health system located in South Bend, Indiana. Memorial's mission statement reflects its commitment to the community: "Memorial is dedicated to improving the quality of life for the people of our community."

Like many hospitals, Memorial has supported a nurse advice call center that uses established protocols to triage patients to get to the right place at the right time. Unlike many hospitals, Memorial has taken this nurse information service to another level.

Ix Applications

In February 2001, Memorial opened the Health Discovery Center as a central access point, or "one-stop shop," for education. The Center is adjacent to the call center and is staffed by call center nurses. Open to the public, the Center provides a reference library of consumer health information as well as computer terminals with Internet access. The Center seeks to bridge inpatient and outpatient care and to support consumers seeking information, referrals, and resources for health and wellness. An advisory board of physicians helped with the planning of the center and also in picking reputable Web sites for consumers to access, including LaurusHealth, JAMA, and Mayo. Nurses are also available by "mouse-call." Community members can e-mail the nurses with questions about health and medical issues; the nurses send back reference material to help consumers make good health decisions.

While most of the traffic into the Center is self-referred, Health Discovery Center staff are actively reaching out to area physicians through the use of preprinted "Rx cards" that doctors can give to patients to encourage them to learn more about their conditions at the Center.

Center staff have also taken their services bedside. Floor staff at the hospital can call upon the Health Discovery Center nurses to arrange for predischarge education and support for patients.

With the creation of the Health Discovery Center and the bedside consults—and the face-to face connections with patients that these generate—Memorial has put a high-touch feel on information therapy.

Clinics

The most powerful information prescriptions are those prescribed by the patient's physician. Physician-prescribed information therapy is what patients want and need most. But can information therapy help the physician and the clinic become more successful?

Among the many factors that influence the success of today's medical clinics, four of the key ingredients are the ability to attract and keep patients; the ability to attract and keep a top-quality staff; information systems that make it easy to deliver high-quality care and get paid for it; and contracts that assure financial success if the clinic cost-effectively delivers high-quality care. An Ix program can help a clinic advance in all four areas.

Patient Recruitment and Loyalty

Information therapy can help attract patients and build strong loyalty both to their physicians and to their clinics. Consumers desire more online interaction with their doctors: while only 3.7 million U.S. adults have e-mailed a doctor's office, 33.6 million more are interested in doing so.[4]

No other physician selection criteria (not even cost, location, or convenient hours) produce such a high response.

With over half of the population already interested and already wanting what information therapy can deliver, the benefit of patient recruitment and increased market share presents the most compelling case for implementing information therapy within a medical clinic.

Staff Recruitment and Retention

Recruiting and keeping physicians, nurses, and ancillary professionals has become a constant struggle for clinics as well as hospitals. Without sufficient staffing, work flow is disrupted, patient and clinician satisfaction declines, and clinic revenues fall. Information therapy helps improve staffing situations in two ways. First, it is an attractive feature for recruiting candidates. Physicians and nurses have gone into their professional fields in part because of their desire to help people. One of the greatest frustrations is the lack of time in most practice situations to help their patients understand their treatment options and what they can do at home for themselves. An Ix program will give doctors and nurses an opportunity to do high-quality, high-value patient education within the time limits of a busy practice. Featuring information therapy in the recruitment communication will be attractive, particularly to those with the highest standards of dedication to their patients and their chosen field of medicine.

Information therapy can also make life easier for clinicians. Work flow is critical to clinic operations, and physicians extending a visit to provide all of the information and education that he or she thinks the patient needs can disrupt work flow. Appointments back up, patient satisfaction levels drop, and physicians' families suffer—all because physicians are trying to do the right thing for patients who need information, support, and guidance. Address the same need with personalized information prescriptions and, presumably, work flow will be facilitated, waiting times will be shorter, and clinicians will get home at more reasonable hours. All that leads to less burnout and greater work-life satisfaction for clinicians as well as increased productivity and reduced staff turnover for the clinic. The patient also gets better information in the process. Everyone wins.

Quality of Care and Reimbursement

Increasingly, clinics must rely on practice management software and information technology both to help their providers practice good medicine and to document what care is provided for billing purposes. Information prescriptions seamlessly launched from the ICD-9, CPT, and NDC codes captured for order entry or billing purposes can activate the patient's potential for improving the quality and outcomes of care. The introduction of handheld devices into the exam room has opened the door to a whole new era of medical practice in which better clinical decisions, fewer medical mistakes, and shared medical decisions will become the norm. Information therapy will be a core part of that new era.

To fulfill the value propositions discussed above, medical clinics can use all seven Ix applications (discussed earlier on page 143). Using an "Information Therapy Assessment for Clinics" similar to that provided in Appendix B, a clinic can begin to identify the low-hanging fruit that an initial Ix program could pursue.

In addition to these value propositions, well-documented and well-qualified information prescriptions may well become reimbursable as either separate or contributory episodes of care. Those clinics already in the business of information therapy will gain a further reimbursement advantage at that time.

Smart Contracts

Information therapy can even play a positive role in a clinic's contract and negotiation activities. Clinics that use information therapy may be able to negotiate lower malpractice costs by improving informed consent and avoiding preventable medical mistakes. They can structure quality incentives with employers or health plans around measures that can be positively influenced by information prescriptions. And they can negotiate direct payment for information prescriptions that meet certain evidence-based, medical appropriateness, timeliness, professional relationship, and documentation criteria.

Virtual Clinics and Physician-to-Patient Portals

Companies like Doctor Goodwell (page 69), WellMed (page 165), and Healinx (page 166) are exploring the frontiers of virtual or e-visits between physicians and their patients. These plans all allow physicians to charge the patient, employer, or health plan for an electronic encounter that responds to a specific patient need. Since the encounter takes place within an information system environment, integrating information therapy into the virtual visit will be relatively easy. Also, because many consumers may prefer an information-rich exchange that gives both their physician's guidance and the evidence-based data behind it, information therapy may become one of the bigger selling points for virtual care.

As with any venture into uncharted territories, virtual clinics are high-stake, high-risk efforts. Their success or failure will be based not only on their value proposition but also on the regulatory environment and market readiness for their services. These plans "call the question" on basic e-health reimbursement issues; their success or failure will have a direct impact on the reimbursement decisions for information therapy.

WellMed
www.wellmed.com

WellMed, of Portland, Oregon, provides a secure online health communication platform that aggregates self-reported health information, integrates it with client systems, and communicates with clients and individuals to guide them in achieving their health-related objectives. The WellMed Health Communication Platform includes three major services:

- The Personal Health Manager, online health management tools for individuals
- Personal Health Insight, tools that help clients analyze Web use patterns
- Personal Health Connect, a secure communication tool used between physicians and patients

Dr. Brad Bowman founded the WellMed clinic in 1993 to help patients identify their health risks and focus on preventive measures. Today, WellMed is dedicated to helping employers and health plans implement their e-health strategies. WellMed has been a leader in working for ethical standards for privacy, security, and quality of online health information.

Ix Applications

WellMed prescribes information based on an individual's personal profile. Instead of expecting the consumer to search for health information that may not be current or relevant, the WellMed Health Communication Platform "pushes" information through a personal health home page, secure messaging, and wireless alerts. WellMed's platform enables health plans and employers to offer high-quality content to members or employees.

Q & A with Craig Froude, WellMed CEO

Q: *What role will information therapy play in WellMed's future?*

A: Information therapy will enable health plans and employers to reduce administrative costs and improve the quality of health information and services delivered to members and employees.

Q: *Your tag line says, "WellMed is the Health Communication Company." What do you mean by that?*

A: WellMed provides a customizable platform that helps organizations connect various constituents of the health care delivery system to improve the delivery of health information and services.

Healinx
www.healinx.com

The mission of Healinx™ is to provide a convenient, clinically structured way for physicians and patients to communicate with one another online.

Founded in 1999, Healinx provides doctors with an interactive Web site through which their patients can securely request a webVisit™ consultation. Patients log into the system either through their physician's Web site or by visiting www.healinx.com.

Ix Applications

The webVisit is an online, nonurgent consultation between a doctor and an established patient. The webVisit guides patients through an interactive questioning process, which then formulates a message to the doctor. Doctors respond to patients by referencing their online health profiles and a database of customizable treatment options. A nurse or other clinical team member can triage and prepare responses to webVisit communications as they would for office visits or telephone calls. Patients can receive self-care information and preventive care reminders, send brief questions, request prescription renewals, and schedule appointments.

A webVisit differs from secure messaging in that the patient messages must be put into a highly structured format. The structure allows greater use of clinical guidelines and algorithms to support the interaction between doctor and patient.

In one pilot program in Silicon Valley, Healinx is providing its webVisit service to selected employees in six high-tech firms. Doctors are paid $20 per online visit, which in some cases is competitive with what doctors "net" from an in-person visit. Additional experiments in what patients or their employers are willing to pay and what physicians will accept will follow as Healinx attempts to demonstrate the value of the webVisit.

In addition to the webVisit, the Healinx service allows physicians to automate preventive care reminders and tailor information to their patient populations.

Healinx seeks to create value for its partners by increasing patient satisfaction and enhancing the efficiency of medical practices.

Electronic Medical Record (EMR) Companies

No strategist in health care can imagine a future health care system without electronic medical records. The case for EMR is just too compelling. A short list of the benefits includes: improved continuity of care; reduced medical errors; vastly improved research capabilities; better patient monitoring and notification capabilities; lower administrative costs; and faster and more accurate billing and collection transactions.

These delights have been in the offing for nigh on 30 years. The adoption of electronic medical records has been remarkably slow, partly because many critics say that the current crop of EMR systems is just not good enough in practice. That criticism no longer holds. Medical practices that do embrace EMR systems now have a significant advantage over those that do not. That advantage will grow over the next few years.

The progression from paper to EMR includes the following steps:

- Physicians use a PDA (personal digital assistant) to look up drugs and doses.

- Physicians place medication orders through a PDA or other device.

- Full order entry is completed on a PDA or other device.

- A full EMR application is integrated with document scanning and chart notes dictation.

Full EMR applications are now available and fully integrated, complete with robust back office functions for billing and quality assurance. Even better, they are now wireless. Products such as Amicore Practice Suite™ have won over a small but growing corps of satisfied clinic clients. While the adoption rate is still slow, those clinics that take the plunge are finding the implementation to be less difficult than they feared and the benefits to be greater than they expected. All the right factors are in place for acceleration in the adoption curve.

Adding Ix capabilities to EMR systems is a no-brainer. An EMR system holds all the triggering information needed to identify the patient's moment in care and to support both physician-prescribed and system-prescribed applications without noticeable change in work flow. Supported applications can include:

- Physician-to-patient information prescriptions prompted by diagnosis and reviewed by the physician at the time of the visit.

- Systems-launched information prescriptions for every new medication order or in advance of refill dates.

- Systems-launched information prescriptions for every lab test ordered or every lab report placed in a patient-accessible record.

EMR companies that pursue that opportunity will find information therapy relatively easy to implement and well received by both physicians and patients. For many physicians it will be the benefit that "sells" them on making the EMR transition.

Amicore
www.amicore.com

Amicore™ develops and delivers information technology and office practices that help to bring back the "joy of medicine." Its focus is on making medical practices healthier by automating, integrating, and transforming practice operations—linking the flow of communications and data from the front desk to the exam room to the back office to outside health care organizations.

Amicore is a privately held physician software and services company formed by a collaboration of Microsoft, IBM, and Pfizer in March 2001. The company later acquired PenChart Corporation, developer of a handheld electronic medical record product that has become a core part of Amicore's "Practice Suite" of clinical and financial products and services.

By offering a complete and integrated set of clinical and financial support services within a dependable, secure, and well-supported hardware and software platform, Amicore hopes to capture a large share of the market for small and mid-sized clinics. Amicore will leverage the reputation and business relationships of its strategic partners (Microsoft, IBM, and Pfizer) to establish itself as a trusted standard that will not vanish with the next dot.com shakedown.

PenChart

PenChart is an automated point-of-care system that documents each clinic visit and enters key information into an electronic medical record. The clinician enters information during the visit into a wireless handheld device the size and shape of a 1-inch-thick clipboard. Notes can be dictated into the PenChart device directly, captured in a digital audio file, and transcribed for review and inclusion into the visit notes. The system can be customized to match the documentation needs and routines of each clinician. With its current customer base, Amicore has a physician adoption rate of over 80 percent.

Secure Messaging

Amicore offers a secure e-mail messaging service that streamlines, tracks, and protects communication and work throughout the practice. The system can send messages directly to the patient.

Ix Applications

Amicore's Clinical Suite now offers patient registration, patient scheduling, medical notes automation, internal messaging, diagnosis coding, and other basic elements of a practice work flow. Each of these elements offers a solid information trigger foundation for launching information prescriptions to patients.

E-Transaction Companies

Another major part of the e-health landscape is the e-transaction processing business. Untold numbers of health care transactions happen each year, and the information systems put in place to manage them represent significant administrative overhead. The high cost, poor efficiency, and high error rates of transaction processing are consistently identified weaknesses of the American health care system. One great promise of e-health is to greatly improve the speed and efficiency of transaction processing and to reduce the management cost of each transaction using Internet-based technologies. Companies like Trizetto, WebMD, and MedUnite have focused on becoming the "place to go" for transaction management in the new e-health era.

The flow of transaction information holds all the triggers needed to implement system-prescribed information prescriptions. Transaction companies that add an Ix service to their offerings will provide their clients yet another value-added reason to shift to their service. The improvements in speed, cost, quality, and service will become too promising to pass up.

Decision-Support Service Companies

Americans make billions of health decisions each year. Decisions about clinic visits, emergency room care, filling medication prescriptions, surgery, testing, mental and physical health—the list is long indeed. Companies that are already offering broader decision-support services will perhaps benefit most from the introduction of information therapy. While information is an essential part of the value chain, information alone does not guarantee value. Value comes with improved decisions. Not only can decision-support companies serve up the core information and decision tools to support a moment in care, but they can also provide nurse care counselors to help the patient work through his or her own case using the information and tools.

Whether through telephone conversation, real-time Internet exchanges, or asynchronous message exchanges, care counselors provide a valuable service in helping callers understand the decision factors and make the decision that is right for them. Satisfaction levels with the services are sky-high. Unfortunately, not that many people call. And those who do call are not always the ones who need it most.

In addition to delivering Prescription-Strength Information and high-quality decision tools, the long-term success of companies in the decision-support business will depend on three factors:

1. How well the company can manage triage calls for immediate decision, low-cost medical services on an Internet-supported, self-triage basis (a lower-cost option than phone calls)

2. How well the company can identify and connect with those patients facing major medical decisions who might not otherwise call them

3. How well the company can encourage self-management of chronic illness through a combination of Internet-based and telephone-based support

Information therapy is key to all three elements of success. Self-prescribed, symptom-based information therapy as described in Chapter 6 is all that is needed for many triage decisions. With good self-assessment guidelines to evaluate their symptoms, most people can reach good decisions about if and how soon they may need care. Encouraging and enabling people to use these self-triage tools first can manage a significant part of the low-yield cases in a cost-effective way.

Information therapy also provides a means for reaching a larger number of people who face major medical decisions. Because EMR and transaction management systems can recognize these moments in care by their information triggers, decision-support information prescriptions can be targeted to everyone who faces a key decision. When it's appropriate and supported by the clinician, care counselors can proactively contact the person to initiate the decision-support exchange.

For disease self-management, information therapy plays many essential roles as well. Information prescriptions on first diagnosis can help recruit people into self-management programs. At periodic points, direct support through nurse care counselors can motivate and encourage continued commitment to the plan. And when information triggers indicate that the moment in care is worsening or relapsing, counselor support can cost-effectively guide the patient to reinforce self-management or treatment decisions. At every stage, the oral support provided by the care counselor on the phone can be backed up with evidence-based Ix prescriptions to the patient either simultaneous with or immediately following the conversation.

Decision-support companies like Health Dialog (profiled on page 70) use information therapy now to enhance their value propositions. As Ix approaches are able to build decision support into the process of care, the value of these services will soar.

Pharmacy Benefit Management (PBM) Companies

Prescription drug benefits have long been among the fastest-rising health care expenditures in America. To control these costs, employers, MCOs, and other groups that provide health benefits are increasingly turning to pharmacy benefit managers (PBMs). PBMs work with patients, pharmacists, physicians, and health plan sponsors to improve the quality of patient care and reduce medical costs. They do this by tracking all prescriptions written by physicians in a health plan with which they've contracted and, in doing so, tracking physician prescribing patterns. They establish formularies (the list of medications that they will reimburse for), administer drug claims, and provide consumer education and disease management programs. Every year PBMs like AdvancePCS, Express Scripts, and Caremark (and over 100 others) serve over 150 million consumers and adjudicate over 1.2 billion prescriptions.[5] That's a lot of medicine.

Advocates credit PBMs with increasing the quality of care; managing costs; bringing a needed focus to disease management; providing necessary patient monitoring, education, and counseling; and a host of other good things. Critics of PBMs are concerned that PBM-related problems, such as compromised patient privacy and too-close-for-comfort relationships with pharmaceutical manufacturers, are compromising patient care.

Friend or foe, industry experts acknowledge that some fairly recent developments in the pharmaceutical landscape will have a notable impact on PBMs. Of these, the growing popularity of direct-to-consumer advertising and the acknowledgement of the extent of medical and prescription errors bear on the need for an Ix approach.

Direct-to-Consumer Advertising

You've seen the ads for prescription medications on television, the Internet, magazines, even on the back of airline luggage tags.

Pharmaceutical companies are spending vast amounts of money to market their drugs directly to the consumer. These investments in advertising have shown a good return on investment. Even though the advertising costs are huge—one estimate was for over $2 billion in 2000—they equal only 2 percent of the total annual expenditure for prescription drugs.[6]

PBMs are challenged by the effectiveness of direct-to-consumer (DTC) advertising. In one recent survey, 19 percent of respondents indicated that they had asked their doctor for an advertised drug. In the same study, 15 percent said they would switch doctors if not given the prescription.[7] Another study has confirmed the impact that DTC advertising has had on consumer buying. According to the Kaiser Family Foundation, nearly 1 in 3 adults has talked to a doctor and 1 in 8 has received a prescription in response to a drug ad.[8]

DTC-advertised drugs fit into roughly three categories, each with a slightly different set of decision factors for the consumer to consider:

1. **Lifestyle drugs.** These offer cosmetic or lifestyle benefits that patients value but that do not impact the long-term outcomes of a serious illness. Examples include Claritin (for allergies), Viagra (for impotence), and Propecia (for hair loss). For the consumer, the decision to purchase these drugs (with a prescription from a physician) may be based on a balance of factors: the out-of-pocket costs involved; the degree that symptoms are bothersome; and the short-term risks the drug may impose.

2. **Prevention drugs.** These are used to reduce the likelihood that disease complications may occur. Examples include drugs for osteoporosis, coronary artery disease, or high cholesterol. With these drugs, an evaluation of the patient's risk for complications from the disease, the risk of taking a long-term medication, and the absolute risk reduction that will occur by taking the medication is important to the decision.

3. **Chronic disease drugs.** These treat diseases such as depression, asthma, or diabetes. The decision here may focus less on the specific drug than on the treatment approach as a whole, including medications, lifestyle changes, and other treatments.

Top Ten DTC Products, 2000

1. *Vioxx®*

2. *Claritin®*

3. *Prilosec™*

4. *Viagra®*

5. *Xenical®*

6. *Paxil™*

7. *Celebrex™*

8. *Propecia®*

9. *Flonase®*

10. *Zyrtec®*

Source: Express Scripts, *2000: Top Developments on the Pharmaceutical Landscape.*[9]

While DTC advertisements are regulated by the FDA to include factual representation of the risks and benefits of each drug, their overall impact is significantly biased toward drug use over other treatment approaches, including self-management behaviors. Using nothing more than the information they now have, plus a current record of consumer e-mail addresses, PBMs could proactively offer people approaching the refill dates for DTC-promoted medications access to unbiased and complete information on both the medication's appropriate use and on other viable treatment alternatives.

Medical and Prescription Errors

New awareness of the high rate of errors involving handwritten medication prescriptions is one of several major factors driving the shift to electronic medication prescription writing using PDAs, wireless tablet PCs, or stationary computer entry devices. In addition to assuring that the prescription is legible to the pharmacist, electronic prescriptions also send instantaneous notification to the PBM. PBM-supported systems can then check the prescription against acceptable dosage ranges for the medication, confirm that the medication does not conflict with other known medications that the patient is taking, and launch an appropriate information prescription. The patient is then able to provide a final level of safety by understanding in advance the medication's approved uses, appropriate doses, look, color, and form.

Over time, Ix prescriptions could become an important part of the PBM service mix. By adding decision support and quality checks, information therapy can help a PBM extend its value, reach, and competitiveness. Employers and health plans alike will value both the consumer service that the PBM-prescribed information will provide and the expected cost-reduction results that may follow wiser decision making about prescription medications.

Disease Management Companies

When pharmaceutical companies, managed care, defined populations, and an aging populace commingled, something new had to come out of the meeting. It did: disease management. Disease management is "a system of coordinated health care interventions and communications for populations with conditions in which patient self-care efforts are significant."[10] Those "conditions" range from asthma to coronary artery disease, depression to diabetes—virtually any chronic illness in which patient self-management behaviors, best practices application, and appropriate use of medications play a part.

The Business of Disease Management

For most successful disease management programs, a common template has evolved:

1. Identify the target population.

2. Confirm that the medication and self-management plans are consistent with evidence-based guidelines.

3. Monitor closely the symptoms, lab values, medication use, preventive services, and other measures, sometimes with help from the patient.

4. Identify and confirm changes in the data that predict a setback in self-management or health status.

5. Use a phone call, nurse visit, physician visit, or other intervention to adjust medication and redirect or reinforce self-management efforts.

6. Educate patients about their conditions so they are better equipped in self-management.

7. Share feedback on performance indicators (at baseline and at periodic intervals) with providers and patients in order to identify areas for improvement.

The value to be achieved from chronic disease management programs is in how well their monitoring and early intervention can keep chronic conditions from flaring into crises. When disease management succeeds, patients have improved quality of life, functionality, and, often, longevity. At the same time, the health care system avoids the high cost of crisis intervention and care.

Disease management reimbursement models include a fixed cost-per-case rate, regardless of severity; capitation rates applied to the entire targeted population; and, increasingly, guaranteed savings plans in which the disease management company is at risk to reduce the overall costs of care for the targeted population. Regardless of the model, information therapy can substantially expand the disease management value proposition. With information therapy, the cost per case goes down, the program's reach within a population expands, and the overall impact on costs is improved.

The data monitoring infrastructure put in place by the disease management company is the ideal source of triggers for launching information prescriptions. The low cost of the information prescription provides a new intervention that can be delivered at the first sign of a data "exception" and before a nurse call or visit can be economically justified. The information prescriptions allow the patient and family to do a better job of self-management and to reduce their need for other, more costly interventions.

CorSolutions
www.corsolutions.com

CorSolutions^SM Medical, Inc., founded in 1994, offers chronic care management services and population-based chronic care management for more than 315,000 individuals affected by chronic diseases, including coronary artery disease, congestive heart failure, chronic obstructive pulmonary disease, diabetes, and asthma. CorSolutions also provides health improvement solutions for over 30 common conditions.

Ix Applications

Through telephone consultation, interactive voice response, home visits, and the company's interactive patient/member Web site (www.eCorsolutions.com), CorSolutions' nurses concentrate on stabilizing and improving patients' health and promoting patient satisfaction and quality of life while reducing unnecessary health care costs. CorSolutions uses the exclusive MULTIFIT^SM approach of physician-directed, nurse-mediated, patient-managed care.

Q & A with Larry Cade, vice president and national marketing director

Q: *What is the company's goal?*

A: To demonstrate outstanding clinical outcomes, improved quality of life for participants, and significant reductions in the overall cost of managing difficult disease-specific populations. We provide a full complement of health improvement programs from prevention and wellness to long-term chronic care. Our intelligence-based approach integrates data analysis, health risk assessment, and predictive modeling. We want to provide our customers with a complete understanding of current and potential health care expenditures. It's a challenge because the U.S. health care industry is established as an acute care model, while we are working to provide care between visits to improve compliance with physician-directed care and support behavioral change for program participants.

Q: *What would you consider to be a home run?*

A: Federal payment for disease management services to providers. This would bring health care improvement into the mainstream.

Beyond Disease Management Toward Health Mastery

The central focus throughout this book has been on using information prescriptions to make better health decisions. That is hugely important and offers many of the low-hanging fruits that will quickly add value to the health care system. Equally important, over the long term, is the potential for information therapy to go beyond discrete decision making around key medical choices and reach a new level called "health mastery."

Health mastery is a personalized approach to health management in which the consumer not only gains understanding of risks and control over day-to-day symptom management but also gains mastery over how the disease impacts his or her life. To reach the health mastery level, information therapy must match in-depth knowledge of the person's moment in care with in-depth knowledge of the individual's preferred learning styles and current level of knowledge.

Chronic diseases are not illnesses to attack, conquer, and move past. They are lifelong illnesses to recognize, accept, and live with. And yet, accepting a disease does not have to mean accepting all of the limitations that normally come with it. With a health mastery approach, people learn to give accommodation to the illness without sacrificing the aspects of their lives that are most important to them.

Profile

HealthMedia, Inc.
www.healthmedia.com

HealthMedia® develops lifestyle management products for distribution via the Internet, print, and other media. These products employ tailored counseling technology that produces health improvement plans unique for each individual.

Dr. Victor Strecher founded HealthMedia in 1998. Much of HealthMedia's approach is based on concepts first developed by Dr. Strecher and his colleagues at the University of Michigan's Health Media Research Laboratory. An impressive body of research has documented substantial benefits from the tailored behavior change approach.

Tailoring, as defined by HealthMedia, means providing advice in a manner that closely approximates a personal counseling session. While HealthMedia's products are similar to counseling, they can reach more people with "in-home" convenience and lower costs. Tailoring implies that the content and sequence of information presented to an individual to support a behavior change is created uniquely for that individual based on information from questionnaires and other sources.

HealthMedia has developed a series of Internet-delivered programs to help people stop smoking, control weight, eat wisely, manage stress, become more fit, and control alcohol consumption. These programs are sold to employers, health care organizations, and others and then recommended to individuals.

Ix Applications

In many ways HealthMedia's tailored messaging approach represents a second generation of information therapy. In the first generation, one might define the right information as information targeted to people facing a common medical decision or challenge. Tailored information differs from targeted information in that it is not only selected to match the person's moment in care but is also created to match the individual's personal preferences and learning styles.

Clinicians and other health professionals can now prescribe the HealthMedia modules in nutrition improvement, smoking cessation, weight management, stress management, and health behavior/risk assessment using the Counselor Assist program. Using the HealthMedia questionnaire in advance of the first counseling session allows the counselor to focus on health improvement planning and goal tracking much earlier in the counseling process.

Governmental and Self-Regulatory Opportunities

The mechanics of information therapy do not inherently lead to greater value. Inaccurate information sent to a patient may be worse than no information at all. Good information sent with the force of a prescription to the wrong person at the wrong time can lead to poor medical decisions. The quality and timing of the information therapy provided is as important as the quality and timing of any other aspect of medical care. Accordingly, government agencies and self-regulatory organizations have both the opportunity and the obligation to expand their current activities to encompass the measurement of quality and outcomes of information prescriptions.

In the U.S., the Agency for Healthcare Research and Quality (AHRQ) is charged with a mission to "support research designed to improve the outcomes and quality of health care, reduce its costs, address patient safety and medical errors, and broaden access to effective services. The research sponsored, conducted, and disseminated by the (agency) *provides information that helps people make better decisions about health care.* [Italics ours.]"[11] AHRQ has an opportunity both to evaluate the effectiveness of information therapy and to promote its use as a good way to close the gap between "what we know and what we do."

The Food and Drug Administration (FDA), the Federal Trade Commission (FTC), and several other parts of the U.S. Department of Health and Human Services (DHHS), including Centers for Medicare & Medicaid Services (CMS, formerly HCFA), Health Resources and Services Administration (HRSA), and the Centers for Disease Control and Prevention (CDC), all have the opportunity to review and adjust their practices in the light of the Ix concept. Hopefully, the right balance will be found that provides strong legal prohibitions of unethical Ix practices without overregulation that stifles innovation or overly burdens administrative costs.

In addition, nongovernmental self-regulatory efforts such as the National Committee for Quality Assurance (NCQA), the Joint Commission on the Accreditation of Healthcare Organizations (JCAHO), and the American Accreditation HealthCare Commission (URAC) have roles to play in information therapy. These groups already do much to monitor and improve the quality of health care services. Extending their activities to cover Ix services is the natural next step. (Note: URAC has already endorsed the 14 principles developed by Hi-Ethics, a coalition of leading e-health companies formed to establish trust among health Web site users.)

Most organizations wishing to offer Ix services to consumers over the Internet should be required to apply for and obtain accreditation and quality monitoring for those services. Exceptions may include efforts by self-help groups to share information among members. Further study is needed to determine how best to monitor and regulate the quality of information therapy directly from physician to patient. Again, the hope is for a balance that provides adequate protection and monitoring without imposing an unnecessary administrative burden.

Hi-Ethics, Inc.
www.hiethics.org

Hi-Ethics™ (Health Internet Ethics) unites the most widely used health Internet sites in an effort to establish and support high ethical standards. Member companies are committed to earning the trust and confidence of consumers by following a set of 14 Hi-Ethics Principles, which can be found at www.hiethics.org. Hi-Ethics is committed to maintaining and enhancing these principles, to ensuring their successful implementation through an industry-developed monitoring program, and to promoting industry self-regulation of health Internet privacy and quality of information for consumers.

The 14 Hi-Ethics Principles cover five general areas of ethical behavior:

1. **Privacy**. The first three principles deal with protecting the privacy of personally identifiable health information submitted to a health Web site. They require the notice of the site's privacy policies and limit the site's ability to use such information unless agreed to by the individual. It also extends the privacy protection to third parties.

2. **Fair trade**. Principles 4, 5, and 6 relate to fair trade practices required of all health Web sites. Principle 4 requires disclosure of the site's ownership. Principle 5 requires that advertising and "sponsored" content be clearly identified, and Principle 6 highlights the limitations placed on promotional offers and discounted services.

3. **Quality of content**. Principles 7, 8, and 9 focus on the quality of the content on health Web sites. Sites are required to post their editorial policies and are prevented from suggesting therapeutic claims without reasonable support. Sites that claim to be based on scientific evidence must disclose who wrote the content. Likewise, dates of creation and update as well as the names and credentials of reviewers are required for some content.

4. **Professionalism**. Principles 10 and 11 require Web sites to clearly describe any professional relationships and to confirm that traditional professional standards remain valid for Internet relationships.

5. **Transparency, limitations, and feedback**. The final three principles require that health Web sites describe themselves clearly to their users and describe their limitations in regards to the practice of medicine. They also call for an easy means to submit feedback or complaints about the site.

URAC/American Accreditation HealthCare Commission
www.urac.org

The Health Web Site Accreditation Program, launched by not-for-profit URAC in 2001, is designed to help consumers identify health Web sites that follow rigorous standards for quality and accountability. The URAC standards are based on the 14 Hi-Ethics Principles. They address the following important concerns: health content editorial process; linking to other Web sites; consumer complaint mechanisms; disclosure of financial relationships; and privacy and security.

URAC's Web site accreditation standards were developed through a process that encouraged broad-based input from consumers, regulators, health care providers, health care organizations, and insurers.

Consumers are able to identify URAC-accredited health Web sites in several ways:

- Every month, URAC issues a national press release announcing the names of all organizations that have achieved accreditation.

- For all accredited Web sites, URAC provides an "accreditation seal" that can be posted on the Web site's home page. This seal links to a URAC Web page that explains the meaning of URAC accreditation.

- The URAC Web site maintains a list of all accredited Web sites, and visitors can click through to those accredited sites.

- The accredited Web site may use its accreditation status in marketing efforts.

Unlike "self-certification" programs, URAC accreditation requires a rigorous third-party audit to assess a Web site's compliance with the standards.

The Health Web Site Standards and other information on URAC is available at www.urac.org.

Q & A with Garry Carneal, president and CEO

Q: *What does a Web site risk by not seeking accreditation?*

A: Accreditation is increasingly important to health care consumers, providers, and regulators, because it demonstrates a commitment to quality. Over the next few years, Web site accreditation will likely become an important part of a company's risk management.

Medical Malpractice Insurers

The $16-billion-a-year medical malpractice business provides yet another approach to self-regulating quality improvement and another avenue for increasing value through information therapy. The rule set for malpractice protection is one of the few approaches to changing physician behavior that seems to work. For better or worse, "cover-your-rear" test regimens, chart notes, and signed releases have all been added to the work flow of medicine to protect against malpractice.

However, it is well established that amount of care and chart documentation are not the critical factors leading to medical malpractice litigation.[12] Patient dissatisfaction is the critical factor. "Breakdowns in communication between physicians and patients lead to patient anger and dissatisfaction and possible litigation. Conversely, effective communication enhances patient satisfaction and health outcomes."[13] Effective communication and overall patient satisfaction provide a level of protection against litigation for physicians, even if they make mistakes and fail to follow the documentation and testing guidelines.[14]

Information therapy is all about improving understanding and communication between doctor and patient. By providing premium discounts to organizations that employ Ix programs as a guard against claims—and by penalizing those that do not—malpractice insurers can change practice patterns. By presenting the right information to the right patient at the right time and by documenting it all electronically, medical malpractice insurers can both improve medical decision making and reduce the risk of successful malpractice suits based on inadequate communication of risks.

The greatest measure of success for medical malpractice insurers has traditionally come from how well they invest their reserves. (Their rates and reserves are heavily influenced by government regulators.) In the future, however, companies that are able to show substantial reductions in malpractice claims experience because of Ix strategies will not only gain the benefit of lower claim payouts but will also grow in market share as clinics and hospitals seek a lower-cost solution.

Large group practices that qualify for experience-rated malpractice insurance rates may be the first to demand Ix programs for their physicians. For them, the improved doctor-patient communication that comes from information therapy will result in both lower costs and improved patient retention and market share.

International Opportunities

This book has been written from a decidedly North American perspective. All of the organizational profiles and most of the work upon which the Ix concepts have been based come from experiences in the United States and Canada. And yet, the human body and the disease process are virtually the same worldwide. With a few exceptions for regionally specific diseases, the same things keep us healthy, make us sick, and help us heal no matter what part of the world we live in. Evidence-based medical knowledge applied to each drug, medical test, surgery, or specific moment in care has universal value.

However, the languages, cultures, financial incentives, and medical practices of the peoples of the world differ greatly. Opportunities abound for both business and governmental efforts that can culturally adapt, translate, and prescribe evidence-based information developed in one country for use in other countries and populations.

Let's think big. Eventually, patient portals, electronic medical records, decision-support services, and other e-health applications will be adapted and adopted internationally. Rich opportunities exist for taking models that work in one country and adapting them to work within the unique characteristics of another. To paraphrase Rene Dubos: think globally, act locally.

Localization, Cultural Adaptation, and Translation of Content

The world body of medical knowledge is immense. Efforts such as the U.K.-based Cochrane Collaboration are establishing a common set of rules for adding to the "evidence base" and allowing for scientific sharing of information.[15] Translation companies and in-country teams for localizing and adapting information are needed in every nation and for every significant population group for whom cultural or language needs are different. This flow of information needs to be multidirectional. Every nation has something to offer in terms of medical knowledge. It is important not to assume that the information flow will only be one-way.

Localization of Information Triggers

System-prescribed information therapy requires that the same attention applied to translating content also be applied to information triggers. The technologies, coding systems, and practice patterns in medicine differ widely from country to country. Each country's information systems must be studied to identify the information triggers that can predict a moment in care. Recoding of the basic content may be needed to create intelligent information that works in a specific medical environment.

Higher Education

Colleges and universities can benefit from recognizing the significance of information therapy and taking early action to contribute to its development. Opportunities fall into two broad categories: student training and health services research.

Student Training

Medical schools must find room in their overly crammed curricula to train medical and nursing students in the how and why of shared medical decision making. Schools that model for their medical students the effective use of information prescriptions will produce graduates more tuned for success with the expectations and needs of the new medical consumer.

Twenty-first-century clinicians need to know how to welcome, develop, and benefit from shared decision-making partnerships with their patients. To do this, they will need to know how to evaluate the quality of information, how to match information prescriptions to the clinical and personal needs of the patient, and how to present an information prescription to maximize patient motivation. Most of all, they will need to learn to think of their patients as partners.

Opportunities for learning more about information therapy are not restricted to those following a clinical career. Schools that teach medical library science, medical record technology, health education, and public health all have an opportunity to collaborate in the creation of a new "certified information therapist" program. Such a program could combine many of the competencies taught in each discipline to produce a professional who could respond to information prescription requests from patients in clinic, hospital, health plan, and open settings.

Health Services Research

Medical schools, nursing schools, and schools of public health have the opportunity to expand their research agendas into the area of information therapy. So many questions present themselves. For example, there are questions of effectiveness and efficiency: What decision-support tools are most effective in helping patients reach fully informed decisions? Which information triggers most efficiently identify or predict the moment in care that a person is approaching? There are unanswered questions about the human interface of information therapy: What tools and techniques enable clinicians to most effectively encourage their patients to use prescribed information? What Ix approaches work best for special populations such as minorities, the elderly, and people with low literacy and other special needs? (We're sure you have some questions of your own . . . The possibilities are endless.)

A New Profession?

Imagine the work of the "information therapist." Just as a certified financial planner helps consumers with their financial planning and goals, the information therapist is trained to coach and assist patients through their medical experiences.

An information therapist would accept information requests from consumers and return recommended links to Internet-available information. The service could range from a low-cost, automated service requiring highly structured input from the consumer to a full concierge service in which the information therapist acts as a private researcher.

Looking Ahead

Prospects for developing and refining Ix goods and services are bubbling up in every corner of the health care system. These opportunities are giving way to practical, consumer-centric solutions to real problems. Using prescriptions of the right information to the right person at the right time, innovators are already improving quality, extending access, and lowering costs across a large range of medical services.

One thing is abundantly clear: Information therapy is only in its infancy. The possibilities for expansion and evolution in scope and effectiveness are limited only by human imagination. Far more opportunities lie ahead.

Reality can be beaten with enough imagination.
Anonymous

8
Health Care in an
Information Therapy Future

Information therapy will change the future of health care. Combined with the forces of evidence-based medicine, Internet-delivered communication, and patient-centered care, information therapy will alter the foundations of health care by redefining both the role of the patient and the role of patient information.

Time for Change

Major conceptual shifts involve both the introduction of new guiding principles and the abandonment of old ones. As in any paradigm shift, those who are most successful under the old rules may have the hardest time championing the new. And only those who embrace the new approaches will thrive.

In the new era of evidence-based, wired, patient-centered care, many of the old and revered tenets of medicine are losing their relevance. Patient compliance and physician autonomy, the tort approach to medical law, the Hippocratic oath—all of these have been cornerstones of the medical profession and health care system as we know them today. But they have also become barriers to the health care system of tomorrow.

The following long-held and often hallowed principles in health care must be put aside in favor of new ideas that support a more active and involved role for the patient.

- **Information as an "extra."** We used to think that health information was "about" care, not a part of care, and thus need not be reimbursed. We now know that good information is central to care and improves medical outcomes. Reimbursement helps ensure that clinicians will provide that information to their patients.

- **Compliance as the preferred model for patients.** We used to think that improving patient compliance would improve health. We now know that passive compliance models result in less active patient involvement in self-care and less successful medical outcomes.

- **Total physician autonomy**. We used to think that every physician was autonomous and could practice on his or her own. We now know that the best medical outcomes occur when clinicians work together in systems that consider evidence-based guidelines and monitor patient outcomes.

- **Tort law as a complete protection for patients.** We used to think that paternalistic tort laws were needed to protect the patient from malpractice and unethical professionals. We now think that shared responsibility for medical decisions, supported by contract law, will result in better outcomes and a fairer sharing of responsibility.

- **The Hippocratic oath as the basis for medical ethics.** We used to think that the Hippocratic oath was the basis for medical ethics. We now recognize that certain aspects of the Hippocratic oath undermine the physician-patient partnership in the new era of health care.

Each of these ideas has served us well at certain times in the past. Each has helped to build the medical profession and health care system as we know them today. Now, each has become an impediment to the health care system of tomorrow. It's time for a change. The new era of health care needs a new set of guiding principles.

Five Rising Stars in Health Care Thinking

1: Information prescribed by a doctor should be reimbursed.

What gets paid for gets done. Clinicians should be reimbursed for prescribing specific information to a patient.

When properly delivered inside a medical practice, information is not just about care; information *is* care. Good information is just as important to good medical outcomes as medical tests, drugs, and procedures. Modest levels of reimbursement for prescribed information would serve to improve the overall quality and lower the overall cost of health care.

Physicians place great value on the information and advice they give to their patients. Patients place great value on the information and advice that they receive. And yet, the health care system places no monetary value on patient information and advice. Physicians who work hard to inform and educate patients about their conditions and treatment choices receive not a penny more than physicians who do nothing more than meet the minimum informed consent requirements.

Because of this value/reimbursement anomaly, the quality of the doctor-to-patient information transfer continues to be abysmally poor, despite the growing availability of technologies that could improve it. The predominant method of delivering patient information uses old-fashioned mouth-to-ear technology. Generally speaking, harried physicians present complicated messages in unfamiliar

Rising Stars in Health Care Thinking

1. *Information prescribed by a doctor should be reimbursed.*

2. *Clinicians and patients should share in medical decisions.*

3. *Medical practice should be evidence-based and objectively measured.*

4. *Medical law should shift from torts to contracts.*

5. *It's time for a new health oath.*

vocabularies to ill and anxious patients. Most of today's knowledge transfer from doctor to patient relies on what the physician remembers (and has time) to tell the patient, what the patient understands, and how much the patient can remember by the time he or she gets home. Unfortunately, so little information makes it through this process that most of the value is lost. There is little confirmation of understanding and few, if any, memory aids for the patient. In a world bristling with both wired and wireless technology, we often don't even use the power of pencil and paper to reinforce memory.

Medicine is rapidly changing to rely more on the patient's involvement in chronic disease self-management and basic medical self-care; the old method of low-yield patient education is no longer tolerable. Prescribing information just as if it were a drug or a test or treatment will result in more-informed and better-trained patients who can provide high-quality home care services and help their physicians reach treatment decisions that better match their needs. Along with the new approach, we need a new reimbursement plan to support it.

Qualifying for Reimbursement

To qualify for reimbursement, medical services must usually meet three criteria: validation, documentation, and appropriateness. The same goes for information prescriptions.

- **Validation.** To be reimbursed, a medical service must be scientifically valid. When information was opinion-based, it could never satisfy the validation criteria. Now, information has the potential to be objectively scored as to its evidence base. The advance of evidence-based medical information satisfies the validation criteria for many information sources. There's work to be done yet: Evidence-based standards must be established and met in order for an information prescription to qualify under the validation criteria.

- **Documentation.** To be reimbursed, there must be a record of how, when, and why a service was delivered. In health care, any addition to the documentation routine or clinic work flow costs money. Documentation entered manually in the patient chart and then manually transcribed for reimbursement purposes costs money. The cost incurred from the slower work flow and record-keeping could price information prescriptions out of range. However, technology makes it possible to include the information prescription without sacrificing time and efficiency. Once a physician order-entry or EMR (electronic medical record) infrastructure is in place, it is relatively painless to add an Ix application. If documentation can then be delivered with no more than a few extra taps on a wireless device, it ceases to be a barrier to reimbursement. Again, there's more work to be done: Documentation standards must be developed and met before widescale reimbursement is possible.

- **Appropriateness.** To be reimbursed, there must be a good reason for a service. No insurer or government program would reimburse heart surgery for people who were not first shown to have heart problems. The same goes for information. Until recently, there has been no practical way to assure that information was appropriately delivered. However, when information prescriptions can be specifically linked to a patient's diagnosis and moment in care, the appropriateness criteria can be easily met.

Restructuring Reimbursement

The Institute of Medicine's 2001 report, *Crossing the Quality Chasm,* has encouraged some efforts to reexamine reimbursement structures: "... to achieve the aims of the 21st century health care system . . . it is critical that payment policies be aligned to encourage and support quality improvement."[1] The report notes that there are disincentives that prevent actions to improve care:

> For example, redesigning care processes to improve follow-up for chronically ill patients through electronic communication may reduce office visits and decrease revenues for a medical group under some payment methods. Current payment policies are complex and contradictory, and although incremental improvements are possible, more fundamental reform will be needed over the long run.[2]

One approach to reimbursement for qualified information prescriptions could come in a redefinition of the formulas for determining whether a clinic visit should be reimbursed as a basic, moderate, or extended visit. Current factors include the number of diagnoses discussed and the number of tests ordered or reviewed. The use of an information prescription could be added as a factor in those formulas.

Alternatively, the American Medical Association, which administers the CPT® (Current Procedural Terminology) codes, could create CPT coding specifically for information prescriptions. Although that approach makes good sense, a major barrier exists to its practical use. Currently, the reimbursement rules allow for visit-based reimbursement or procedural-based reimbursement for a service or encounter—either one or the other, but not both. The clinician must choose which approach to follow. Because the value of an information prescription CPT code is likely to be small, it is unlikely that a physician would ever submit that code rather than a clinic visit or procedure code unless an exception to the "either/or" rule were allowed.

Need proof that reimbursement for information works? Here's another thought: The Centers for Medicare & Medicaid Services (CMS) could fund pilot programs to test the impact of information prescription reimbursement on both the quality of medical outcomes and the overall cost of care.

Consideration of reimbursement for qualified information prescriptions is a part of a broader reimbursement alignment effort being undertaken by the eHealth Initiative (eHI), a developing trade association for e-health companies.[3] The eHI reimbursement committee is charged with supporting policy development in the areas of technology-aided virtual clinic visits, physician-patient e-mail, and interactive disease management systems along with information prescriptions.

Again, what gets paid for gets done. Good information is critical to good care, and reimbursement is critical to the delivery of good information.

2: Clinicians and patients should share in medical decisions.

The "doctor-knows-best" approach to medical care used to make sense. Not so long ago, a person's best outcomes came from picking a good doctor and then trusting him to prescribe the right care. The patient's role was to do just what he or she was told—nothing less and certainly nothing more.

Times have changed. "Doctor knows best" has evolved to "the doctor is your best partner." Why involve the patient to such a high degree? First, the science of medicine has grown faster than any single physician's ability to keep up. Even if a physician could spend 8 hours a day, 7 days a week, reading medical studies and attending continuing medical education classes, the advance of medical knowledge would soon outpace his or her efforts. Physicians do well with the problems that they see and deal with frequently. However, catching the rare diagnosis is often a matter of whether or not the physician was lucky enough to see a recent article in a specialty or subspecialty medical journal. Even among common problems, there are significant variations in treatment by physician, by clinic, and by geographic region of the nation. Blind trust in doctors' orders becomes acceptable to fewer and fewer patients when their treatments and outcomes are known to depend so much on the luck of the draw.

The compliance model has been further unsettled by the emergence of the informed patient. Active and informed consumers have discovered that they can improve the outcomes of their care by learning more about their diseases and their treatment options. (And, certainly, the 24/7 health Internet feeds that interest.) Active patienthood has been reinforced by success stories that demonstrate, time and again, that the best medicine is practiced when patients and their doctors work together.

When patient and doctor arrive at decisions jointly, the notion of compliance is replaced by that of adherence. Patients elect to honor and to follow their treatment plan. By definition, to be compliant means to acquiesce or give in to requests or demands. As such, compliance is the antithesis of active partnership or empowerment in health care. To adhere, on the other hand, is to give support to a plan. Aside from the semantics, there is a critical shift in authority and responsibility from clinician to patient. As discussed in Chapter 7, a patient-centered approach to care is being adopted by leading hospitals as a major part of their efforts to reduce medical errors.

Lots of effort has been expended on helping doctors improve patient compliance, and with good reason. The consequences of noncompliance—not taking prescribed medications, for example—are poor outcomes, greater risks, and greater costs. But if compliance worked well in the old model, shared decision making and adherence to the common plan should work even better today.

3: Medical practice should be evidence-based and objectively measured.

The first randomized clinical trial was not completed until the 1950s. Just a half-century later, thousands of articles based on randomized clinical trials are added to the medical literature each year. Little by little, these trials are telling us what works in medicine and what does not. The cumulative knowledge from these trials goes far beyond the clinical experience of any single physician.

That is not to say that the physician's experience is of any less value. Physicians must interpret evidence-based guidelines in light of the specific situation of the patient. To do that requires both the clinician's expertise and an ability to consider the patient's values and preferences. Clinical experience and patient preferences must likewise be applied in consideration of the medical evidence.

What does this have to do with information therapy? A lot. Information therapy will prescribe evidence-based medical information based on the patient's clinical status. The physician must then help the patient reach medical decisions that are informed by the information they receive plus insights from the clinician's experience and patient's values.

The monitoring of clinical outcomes by clinician, facility, and region is also an important part of health care in the future. The primary purpose of outcome tracking is to improve the system and to improve the health of the patients in it. Eventually, outcome tracking leads to an improved information base for everyone.

4: Medical law should shift from torts to contracts.

Medical malpractice law is built on the concept of torts. What is tort law?

> Torts are wrongs that the law recognizes as grounds for a lawsuit. Torts include an intentional slap in the face, a negligent automobile accident, medical malpractice and even environmental pollution. All tort actions begin when a person commits some type of harm to another that the law says constitutes a legal injury. The injured party has what is known as a "cause of action" that can be pursued in a court of law. Tort damages can

be either compensatory or punitive. Compensatory damages are aimed at paying the harmed party for the value of his or her loss, while punitive damages are money damages that are sought to punish the wrongdoer. Punitive damages have no relation to the actual value of the harm done. They are set by the jury or court to simply punish the wrongdoer and serve as a future deterrent to hopefully prevent the same harm from being done again.[4]

The application of tort law in health care generally assumes an ignorant and unprotected patient being served by an educated and authoritative professional. The professional must choose wisely in prescribing and administering treatments and act within professional standards to avoid claims of malpractice. If the physician makes a mistake—"commits some type of harm"—then he or she is liable.

Perhaps we are asking too much of physicians and too little of consumers of health care. As consumers gain access to more medical information and participate more as partners in medical decision making, contract law may better replace tort law.

What is contract law? Simply put, contract law is the law that governs contracts. A contract is an agreement between two or more people that creates an obligation to do, or not do, something. The three factors necessary to create a contract are offer, acceptance, and consideration (recompense). One party must make an offer, the second party must accept the offer, and consideration must be exchanged. The agreement creates a legal relationship of rights and duties. If the agreement is broken (breached), then the law provides remedies.[5]

Under contract law, two parties—in this case, the doctor and the patient—agree as equals to an action. When the patient has access to high-quality information about his or her options and plays an active role in the treatment decision, he or she should also bear a greater share of the responsibility for the outcomes. The clinician's legal burden is correspondingly less.

We are not saying that this will happen overnight. Changes in the legal system are, appropriately, wrought slowly over a long period of time, and some elements of tort law should never be abandoned. Licensed professionals must continue to have an obligation to practice

Please note:

See Appendix A beginning on page 213 for an in-depth discussion of informed consent, malpractice, privacy, and other legal issues in information therapy.

in their patients' best interests, and we must guard against falling into a "blame the victim" mentality. But with shared decision making will eventually come an increased level of shared legal responsibility for the actions that are taken and the outcomes that result.

5: It's time for a new health oath.

The Hippocratic oath is considered with pride as a foundation for every physician's sense of professionalism. Reportedly, it is used by 98 percent of medical schools in the U.S. and Canada, generally as part of their graduation ceremonies.[6]

The original Hippocratic oath is attributed to Hippocrates, a fourth-century Greek physician and medical teacher whose collection of medical writings included a code of principles for the teachers of medicine and their students. The oath consists of two major parts. The better-known and often-referenced second part of the oath includes the physician's pledge to offer only beneficial treatments, to prescribe "no deadly drug," and to live an exemplary personal and professional life. That pledge has become the foundation of medical ethics and professionalism in medicine.

The first part of the code, however, is focused on the relationships between the teacher and student of medicine. Included in this section is the following statement:

> I will impart a knowledge of the Art to my own sons, and those of my teachers, and to disciples bound by a stipulation and oath according the law of medicine, but to none others.[7]

Why Hippocrates placed a restriction on sharing medical knowledge is unknown. We do know that Hippocrates charged his students a fee.

Perhaps requiring secrecy was his way of preserving the proprietary value of his information. A millennium later, the concealment of medical information is no longer acceptable. There should be no restrictions placed on who shall have access to medical knowledge. As long as the privacy of individuals is protected, the availability of medical knowledge should be and is open to all.

California-based pediatrician Alan Greene, MD, who pioneered early physician Web sites with the creation of drgreene.com, has brought attention to this anachronism in the Hippocratic oath in numerous presentations and articles. Greene proposes that the oath be reinterpreted for the new era of care. His proposed "Millennium Health Oath" provides no support for secrecy in medicine (except in the area of privacy protection) and includes the following strong enforcement for shared decision making:

> I will provide also the means for people to evaluate that which I recommend and the means to make their own health decisions with the benefit of my expertise and thoughtful counsel.[8]

Dr. Greene shares with hundreds of thousands of physicians a passion for teaching patients all that they "shall wish to learn." For many physicians the "art" of medicine has been lost within the bureaucratic battles of managed care, federal regulations, and complex technology. In the midst of the medical-industrial complex they find simple solace in the pleasure of sharing their skills and knowledge with patients who want to learn.

While Dr. Greene's version of the oath may never catch on within the medical schools of the world, it has captured the truth of the current age and holds the wisdom for professional success in the new era.

Please note:
See pages 234 and 235 for the full text of the Hippocratic oath and the proposed Millennium Health Oath.

An Evolved Role for Physicians: Navigator and Coach

Through all of these changes, the physician will remain critical to the success of the health care system and to the health of all patients. Still, the physician's role will change. New thinking about the patient's role in every aspect of care calls for reciprocal changes in the physician's role.

In primary care, it is clear that the real primary care provider is either the individual patient or a caregiving family member. No primary care system will succeed without integrating the role of the patient/family member into the basics of care. The physician's role is no less important and in no way expendable—the one-to-one relationship with a trusted physician will still be critical. However, the assumption that care needs to be delivered through discrete clinic visits is being replaced by information technology solutions that extend the reach of the clinician beyond the clinic walls.

In chronic disease, it is clear that self-management activities performed daily by the patient with the support of others is the most critical part of disease management. Again, no plan will find success without fully engaging the patient and the family as a part of the provider team. Physicians using secure messaging and automated monitoring will be able to fine-tune medications and track progress without putting undue strain on clinic facilities and practice hours.

Many forward-thinking health care leaders have used an airplane analogy to illustrate the new doctor-patient relationship. In the old model, the physician was the pilot and the patient a passenger in the plane. In the new model, the patient is the pilot and the physician is the navigator and, often, the flight instructor. Using his or her experience, insights, and knowledge, in addition to any help provided by medical guidance systems, the physician tells the patient where the plane is, what mountains surround it, when storms might pose a problem, and what flight paths to take to avoid them. With that help from the physician, the patient has the choice of either making the final decisions or delegating them back to the physician. The physician must be ready to take over the controls again at any such moment.

With good coaching, good information, and supportive communication technology between physician and patient, the amount of care that the patient and family can provide for themselves is almost without limit. True, we don't expect (or want) manuals for do-it-yourself brain surgery to proliferate. There will always be a great need for skilled professionals to do what only they are trained to do well. We do expect, however, that the legal doctrine of informed consent will be expanded to support higher degrees of control, authority, and responsibility for every patient. The shift, we think, will usher in a more productive and satisfying era of medicine for physicians and patients alike.

Predictions for an Information Therapy Future

- Every medical visit, test, drug, or treatment will trigger an information prescription.

- Every inpatient will get new information prescriptions with each new order entry.

- Information prescriptions will be defined as a medical service and reimbursed.

We have a high level of confidence that these predictions are accurate. We are less sure of their timing. Much will depend on how quickly the wireless, electronic medical record, and order-entry infrastructure reaches mainstream medicine. Once those systems are in place, the consumer demand for and organizational benefits from information therapy will push wide-scale implementation quickly.

Information therapy not only redefines information as a part of medicine—it also redefines the role of the patient as a partner in medical decision making and a full member of the provider team. Information is care. The patient is on the provider team. The rest is easy.

The greatest untapped resource in
health care is the consumer.
Vernon Wilson, MD

The Healthwise Story:
The Evolution of an Idea

As told by Don Kemper, founder, chairman, and CEO

Imagine, if you will: The year is 1970. I'm a 24-year-old lieutenant in the U.S. Public Health Service. I have a degree in engineering science and am halfway toward a master's degree in systems engineering. And I have all the arrogance you would expect of a young engineer.

My job in the USPHS is to apply systems thinking to health care. So far, my focus has been on looking at hospitals as whole systems (that is, don't just look at the laundry or the pharmacy as separate units—all the parts must work together). In 1970 this was fairly innovative.

Now imagine me sitting down in a large government auditorium to listen to my boss's boss's boss, Vernon Wilson, MD. At that time Dr. Wilson was the Assistant Surgeon General in charge of the Health Services and Mental Health Administration (HSMHA, affectionately known as Hiss Ma Ha). Medical technology was all the rage. The government was pushing the creation of CCUs and ICUs across America. Futurists were promising that hospitals would soon have computerized information systems coordinating every aspect of care. Clearly, this was a time for systems engineering, and I was expecting the talk to be focused along these lines. Instead, Vernon Wilson delivered a different message. His theme was simple: "**The greatest untapped resource in health care is the consumer.**"

I sat up and listened carefully. Things started to click for me:

- "The patient is a part of the system."

  If the consumer is the greatest untapped resource in health care, the consumer (the patient) is a part of the system.

- "Why not improve the system by making the patient smarter?"

  I had a little baby at home at the time, and someone had given me a copy of *Dr. Spock's Baby and Child Care* to make me a smarter parent. Surely this approach could work for other things too.

- "Why not develop a Dr. Spock for the whole family to tap the consumer resource?"

- "Why not give the book to every family in America to help them make good health decisions and to practice good health care at home?"

- "Why not use the Office of the U.S. Surgeon General to help change the role of the consumer from that of a patient to that of a partner?"

Wow! This was exciting! The next morning I presented the plan to my boss. She laughed. And while she didn't stop me from talking to others, I could never get senior-level support for the idea. I left the Public Health Service a year later, somewhat battered and without having made any progress toward tapping the consumer resource of which Dr. Wilson had spoken.

Still, that core idea—tapping the consumer resource in health care—stuck with me.

A Second Chance

After finishing my systems engineering studies at Georgia Tech, I entered an MPH program at Berkeley. Under the mentoring of Henrik Blum, C. West Churchman, and other professors, I learned to apply the systems approach to health planning. A vision of patient-centered care began to emerge.

In 1972 I took a job in Boise, Idaho, to work with Health Systems, Incorporated, which was funded by the National Center for Health Services Research. Our assigned mission was to "rock the health care boat" for the 3-year period of the grant and then get out. In rocking the boat, we introduced Idaho's first EMT training, first nurse practitioner training, and first health maintenance organization.

My new boss, Doug Mitchell, also let me dust off the old idea. In 1973 we developed and taught a course through the Boise Community Schools Program called "The Parent's Role in Health Care." Sixteen moms came to a local school once a week for 12 weeks (!) to learn how they could better deal with colds, flu, headaches, backaches, and the like. They enjoyed the class. We were encouraged to go further.

In 1974 we created a television show and community program called "Common Sense: Common Health." We organized 24 viewing groups from PTAs and church groups in Boise who came together once a week to watch a 30-minute show and then call into a radio program for questions and answers with a different health professional every week. Topics included respiratory problems, headaches, backaches, and other common ailments. We were further encouraged by consumer responsiveness.

In 1975, as Health Systems, Incorporated was winding down, we spun off the health education projects into a new nonprofit 501(c)(3) organization that we named Healthwise, Incorporated. Our mission is "to help people make better health decisions."

Early Grant Support: 1976-1990

With an initial grant from the Kellogg Foundation to develop the materials and a follow-up grant from the National Center for Health Services Research to evaluate the approach, Healthwise launched what has now been a 26-year effort to help people make better health decisions.

- We wrote the first edition of the *Healthwise® Handbook* in 1976. (It is now in its 15th edition with over 20 million copies in print.)

- We created the Healthwise Self-Care Workshops based on what we had learned from the earlier efforts and sold instructional materials to employers, hospitals, community groups, churches—anyone who wanted to create smarter health care consumers.

- Through evaluation studies, we showed that the people who attended the workshops actually had lower health care costs.

- We developed "Help Yourself to Health," a workshop program designed to empower participants in the USDA's WIC (Women, Infants, and Children) program to make better nutrition decisions.

- With funding from the Centers for Disease Control and Prevention, we developed "Growing Younger," a workshop program to encourage older adults toward better fitness, nutrition, stress management, and self-care behaviors.

- Through a grant from the Meyer Charitable Trust, we developed "Growing Wiser," a workshop program to encourage older adults toward new thinking about wisdom and vital aging and to build skills to deal with memory, chronic pain, depression, loss, and other concerns.

We also began to sell our books, videotapes, and instructor guides in increasing numbers to managed care organizations, hospitals, and health departments. Still, grants covered the bulk of our modest expenses as our staff size grew slowly from 4 to 12 people over a 14-year period.

During these years Healthwise developed an increasing national and international reputation for leadership in medical self-care and health empowerment programs. We sponsored two national conferences (in 1977 and 1979) to help others to understand and succeed in applying the concepts of empowerment and self-care to the populations they were serving. And we served on the boards of organizations like the National Wellness Institute, the National Primary Care Association, and the American Society on Aging to extend our ideas into related organizations.

The "Mainstreaming" Years: 1990-2001

In 1990 a single event marked a sea change in the focus and path of Healthwise. Health Net, a California-based managed care organization, had all but accepted our proposal to sponsor Healthwise workshops for 10,000 of their members through their contracting employers. To seal the deal, they asked that Healthwise make a final presentation of the plan to their senior staff, including Roger Greaves, their CEO. Molly Mettler made the trip. (Molly is my spouse, my coauthor, and senior VP for Healthwise.) But she left with a radical new plan to present. Instead of trying to "close" on the workshop proposal, Molly suggested that each Health Net family that did not have a copy of the *Healthwise Handbook* was at a disadvantage.

Roger Greaves liked what he heard. In addition to the workshop plan, Health Net committed to distributing 300,000 copies of the *Healthwise Handbook*—one to every Health Net subscriber. We dubbed the shift from the workshop to the home as the "**mainstreaming**" of self-care and set about to make that happen in other organizations. Over the next 11 years, Healthwise contracted with eight of the ten largest health plans in America. Many, like Kaiser Permanente and Group Health Cooperative, have given a copy of the *Healthwise Handbook* to each of their subscribing families. By the end of the twentieth century, there was a book in one out of every ten American homes. We know from research studies that once the book is in the home, it is used, on the average, seven times a year. So, our information was being turned to an average of 70 million times a year. We were clearly making a difference.

The Healthwise® Knowledgebase: The 100-Year Project

The revenues from book sales gave Healthwise the resources to extend the vision of helping people make better health decisions. In 1990 we started planning the creation of the Healthwise Knowledgebase. From the start, the vision of the Knowledgebase has involved three key phrases:

- **All of Medicine**—Finding the best information on every medical problem

- **Decision-Focused**—Organizing the information around health decisions

- **Consumer-Friendly**—Translating the information into terms that most people understand

Undaunted by counsel from friends and colleagues who advised that the job was too big, we dubbed it the "100-year project" and started to build it.

By 1994 the Knowledgebase was starting to take shape as an electronic product that nurses could use to answer patient questions. It was set up on computers in nurse call centers. It worked. Prior to that, nurses relied on their clinical experience and an assortment of index cards to respond to questions. The new Knowledgebase allowed the nurses to quickly look up the caller's problem and respond with the help of the Knowledgebase's in-depth, decision-focused information.

The Healthwise goal was to get that information to as many consumers as possible and as directly as possible. When CD-ROM technology reached the consumer, we thought that might be the best path, despite our worry that CD-based information might soon be out of date. The emergence of the Internet changed that: we knew it held great potential for our new mission.

Evidence-based medicine caught our eye early. We were soon researching every PORT (Patient Outcomes Research Team) study and outcomes research report released. We developed our national medical review board specifically around those specialists at the front of the evidence-based medicine movement. We developed a strong commitment to fully documenting all information presented.

We also came to realize that if information doesn't help people make better health decisions, it doesn't really help. We set to work creating Healthwise "Decision Points," which are consumer guides to making specific decisions about medical tests and treatments. Since "decisions" in the broad sense also includes decisions about changing health behaviors, we developed a long series of "Actionsets" to help consumers focus on the health behavior changes most effective for improving their condition.

While our content strength was in "deep" written content, we began to enhance it through multimedia presentation. To assure that the content was consumer-friendly, we brought in national experts on readability to train our writers and editors. The result was the creation of the "Healthwise style," which permeates all of our health information. Through the uses of bullets, plain language, and a direct approach, we found we could present complex medical issues in a way that most people could understand.

By 2001 our Healthwise Knowledgebase was available on more than 400 different Web sites. It had also been picked up internationally and made available by the Ministry of Health for British Columbia, Canada; by the British United Provident Association, the United Kingdom's largest insurer; and by a number of clients in South Africa.

Healthwise as a Technology Company

As the 1990s progressed, it became clear that to succeed in its mission, Healthwise would need to become a technology company. Technology is essential to us in three areas: document management, content delivery, and content intelligence.

Document Management Technology

The *Healthwise Handbook* covers about 200 health topics in about 350 pages. The Knowledgebase covers thousands of topics in thousands of pages. That's a lot of information to manage. In response, Healthwise has developed an authoring and document management system that networks in-house and remote authors and reviewers. But the basic task is nothing compared with the challenges of maintaining customized versions to meet the needs of large managed care organizations and other large clients across three continents. As the Knowledgebase is translated into other languages, the demands on document management technology will continue to expand.

Content Delivery Technology

We've come to learn that there is no single technology standard that works for every client. Since the Knowledgebase gains its greatest value when launched within other enterprise-wide applications or more global-purposed Web sites, we had to match our delivery with many different needs. Currently, Healthwise makes content deliveries to client Web sites in LAN, HTML, and XML formats as well as through an ASP model Web site that Healthwise hosts. Pursuit of the elusive universal platform continues.

Content Intelligence Technology

By the end of the 1990s, Healthwise had realized the power of embedding "intelligent tags" into the content and providing content indexing that would allow for an automatic matching of content to structured medical languages and medical codes, such as ICD-9 diagnosis codes or CPT®-4 procedure codes. These tags require constant expansion and modificiation as coding systems are updated and new terminology systems are added to the content.

Ethical Leadership

Healthwise has also worked hard to raise the bar for ethical practices on the health Internet.

Healthwise was a charter member of **Hi-Ethics** (Health Internet Ethics), a coalition of large health Web sites that work together to create a standard of ethical principles that all health Web sites are encouraged to follow. (I was privileged to serve as the founding chairman and president of Hi-Ethics.) The 14 Hi-Ethics Principles have been widely acclaimed and are used as the basis for the URAC Health Web Site Accreditation Program. In December 2001 Healthwise was among the first 13 health Web sites to receive accreditation from URAC and the right to display the URAC Health Web Site Accreditation Seal.

The Center for Information Therapy: 2002 and Beyond

If building the Knowledgebase is a 100-year project, fully developing information therapy may take a millennium. We established the Center for Information Therapy in January 2002 to advance the art, science, and practice of information therapy. The Washington, D.C.-based center is a separate division of Healthwise charged with five objectives:

1. **Innovation.** To cosponsor with clinics, hospitals, and health plans innovative Ix solutions in prevention, visit prep, triage, self-care, self-management, decision support, and end-of-life care.

2. **Communications.** To write articles, present talks, sponsor conferences, and organize electronic communities to share ideas, progress, and enthusiasm among Ix innovators and future players.

3. **Evaluation.** To convene researchers and funding organizations to set the Ix research agenda, establish common outcome and process measures, and assure broad dissemination of evaluation results.

4. **Outreach.** In partnership with Healthwise, to make substantial and unusual efforts to extend the value of Ix prescriptions to the uninsured and underserved.

5. **Policy.** To write position papers, provide testimony, and encourage debate on public and private policies leading to the support and reimbursement of information therapy.

The Information Therapy Commission

While the fiduciary responsibility for the Center for Information Therapy rests with the Healthwise Board of Directors, its policy work will be set by the Information Therapy Commission. The 11-member commission is charged with helping the Center set priorities among the many potential opportunities for innovation, communication, evaluation, and research. The commissioners include prominent leaders across a broad spectrum of health care.

Full-Circle: Where Will the Story End?

This story began as a vision in 1970. While the Healthwise tale has taken many turns along the way, it has always remained true to the basic ideas:

• The patient is part of the system.

• We can improve the system by helping people make better decisions.

• We can help people make better decisions by providing accurate, up-to-date, and clinically relevant information to everyone.

Now that we have added "the right information to the right person at the right time" as a guiding theme, Healthwise and the new Information Therapy Commission are set on achieving a second set of basic ideas:

• Prescribe relevant, evidence-based information as a part of every medical service.

- Support shared decision making as part of every treatment plan.

- Encourage evidence-based self-management as a key part of every chronic care plan.

The next pages of the Healthwise story will focus on both sets of ideas. The Healthwise Knowledgebase will grow to provide decision-support information on every health decision. The Center for Information Therapy will extend the art, science, and practice of prescribing information as part of every moment in care.

The Healthwise story has come a long way from its birth over 30 years ago. The most interesting part of the story has yet to be written.

Legal Issues in Information Therapy

Disclaimer: We are not attorneys, and this appendix does not include legal advice. It is a collection of remarks on informed consent, medical malpractice, and privacy and how information therapy relates to them. Because health law differs in every state, specific legal interpretations and advice should be sought from locally practicing attorneys.

Very little in American medicine can be done without careful consideration of the legal ramifications. Three legal issues most likely to become factors in implementing information therapy include informed consent, medical malpractice, and privacy/confidentiality.

Informed Consent

Informed consent is a fundamental principle of medical law. The purpose of this doctrine is "to give the patient sufficient information so that he or she has the opportunity to make a knowledgeable and informed decision about the use of a drug or device in the course of treatment."[1] With clear exceptions for people not of sound mind or in emergency situations, a person has the right to decide what becomes of his or her body. A physician who fails to provide the patient sufficient information to make a knowledgeable and informed treatment decision is negligent of a professional duty to do so and is considered in breach of the standard of disclosure.[2]

How much information does a physician have to provide to meet the standard? *Legal Medicine* offers a robust definition of what is required:

> To give an informed consent to medical treatment, a patient should be told his or her diagnosis, the differential diagnosis, the nature of the diagnosis, the nature of the therapeutic procedure to be performed, the material risk associated with his or her care and management, the prospect of success of the treatment (i.e., the prognosis or expectations), and the detail of alternative courses of treatment that are available. The physician has the duty to inform the patient of the adverse consequences of any proposed treatment or procedure so as to enable the patient to make an intelligent decision about whether or not to consent to the treatment. This duty is particularly compelling when the recommended treatment includes a type of elective surgery and the probability of the risk might dissuade a person from submitting to the treatment.[3]

Courts have established four elements of the informed consent requirement:[4]

1. The physician should explain the nature of the procedure, treatment, or disease.

2. The physician should present realistic expectations of the recommended treatment and the likelihood of success.

3. The patient should know what reasonable alternatives are available and what would likely happen without treatment.

4. The patient should be told of any specific risks that could likely affect the patient's decision to accept or reject a recommended treatment.

How Information Therapy Will Support Informed Consent

While these four elements of informed consent are universally agreed upon in theory, they have not been consistently followed in practice. Information therapy could change that. Specifically designed to help patients understand their health problems and the potential courses of action, information prescriptions provide a solid basis for the informed consent requirement. They also leave a well-documented record of the informing action. Obtaining informed consent should become much easier to do.

Medical Malpractice

Medical malpractice—"any professional misconduct that encompasses an unreasonable lack of skill or unfaithfulness in carrying out professional duties"[5]—also needs to be considered in the context of information therapy. To win a medical malpractice case against a physician, a plaintiff must prove each of these four following elements:[6]

1. **Duty.** It must be shown that the physician had a "duty" to perform a professional service with the same degree of skill, knowledge, and care as a reasonable and prudent physician in his or her same specialty at the same time. Generally, this means that the plaintiff must prove that a "standard of care" exists relative to the malpractice claim.

2. **Breach of duty**. It must be shown that the physician did not comply with the standard of care in some clear and measurable way.

3. **Causation**. It must also be shown that the breach of duty was the legal or proximate cause of an injury or harm to the patient. Generally, proving a breach of duty as a contributory or even primary cause of injury is not enough. The breach must be proven to be the sole cause of an injury to win a ruling under most laws.

4. **Damages**. It must be shown that the injury created damages to the patient.

How Information Therapy Can Reduce the Risk of Medical Malpractice

Information therapy can reduce a physician's exposure to malpractice in three ways. First, by meeting the physician's professional obligation to obtain informed consent, the use of information prescriptions eliminates the neglect of informed consent as a possible cause of a malpractice claim. Secondly, because information prescriptions can provide in-depth information to patients about their treatment, they allow patients to catch medical errors or potential medical errors before any harm is done. The most important impact of information therapy on malpractice will most likely come because of improved patient-physician relationships. Information therapy that fully informs patients about their conditions, recommended treatments, and alternatives will help build patients' trust in their physicians.

When a patient is informed and shares in the treatment decision, he or she is less likely to file suit, even if the outcome is not as expected or desired.

Privacy and Confidentiality: Protecting Personally Identifiable Health Information

Information therapy is all about the use of individually identifiable health information to target specific Prescription-Strength Information to specific consumers. Without the use of highly private and confidential material, information therapy would be nothing more than "general-information-to-no-one-in-particular-at-no-specific-time." No name, no diagnosis, no identifiers, no record? No good. However, any abuse of consumer confidentiality and trust will sink Ix innovations utterly and completely.

The electronic distribution of medical records, service requests, test results, and every other element of medical information will become the norm in twenty-first-century health care. Because the information prescriptions sent to a specific person for a specific problem meet the definition of personally identifiable medical information, they must be administered with the same level of security protection as any other part of the patient's medical record. It's a basic requirement for doing business.

So, who's paying attention? The enactment of the Health Insurance Portability and Accountability Act of 1996 (HIPAA) has raised the bar on the level of protection clinicians, hospitals, and health plans must provide for their patients' and members' medical records and related information. Other federal and state legislation, as well as the self-regulatory efforts of URAC (www.urac.org) and NCQA (www.ncqa.org), pays close attention to privacy protection.

The two basic ethical rules regarding the use of personally identifiable health information are as follows:

1. Health-related personal information should be used only for the purposes for which a reasonable consumer would expect them to use it or as agreed to by the consumer.

2. Health-related personal information should not be disclosed to an unrelated third party or for unrelated purposes without first obtaining the explicit "opt-in" consent of the consumer.

While HIPAA and COPPA (Children's Online Privacy Protection Act of 1998) both provide reams of guidelines, interpretations, and regulations expanding on those rules, the basic principles are quite clear. How, then, do they apply to information therapy?

Is it permissible for a physician to send an information prescription to a patient without the patient's request? Yes, unless the patient has explicitly asked not to receive such information. Most reasonable consumers would expect their physicians to be able to send them information if the physician thought it might help.

It is generally expected for a physician to report personal health information to a health plan so that the health plan will pay the patient's bill. Is it, then, also reasonable and expected for the health plan to use that same information to trigger the transmission of an information prescription to the patient that might help him or her to manage the health problem involved? Here the need for an explicit opt-in approval from the member may be more open to interpretation. Most consumers might expect such supportive action from their health plans, but certainly not all. Definitely, the health plan would be on safer ground if the plan explicitly described that service in the policy information that is given to each subscriber. Some plans may choose to follow an even safer approach of asking for opt-in approval within the plan application process.

Is it ethically or legally allowable for a physician to send a copy of an information prescription to the spouse or friend of the patient? Not without a signed consent from the patient, a medical power of attorney, or an emergency situation preventing the patient from providing consent. Any sharing of information with others requires the patient's explicit approval. Specific exceptions are made for the parents of minor children or when medical conditions prevent the patient from providing such approval.

Underlying these basic questions is an increasingly important obligation to keep all personally identifiable patient information tightly secure. The current permeability of e-mail suggests a much needed shift toward secure messaging systems. With secure messaging, a patient receives an e-mail notifying him or her of a message waiting on a password-protected site. The patient then must use his or her password to gain full access to the information.

In the years ahead, privacy, confidentiality, and security issues will continue to loom large and affect the reach of information therapy via direct doctor-patient communication and also via health Web sites. In addition to meeting all HIPAA regulations, the following guidelines may be useful in preparing an Ix program for health Web site accreditation.

- Organizations must disclose to users what information is collected about users and how it is used; to whom personally identifiable information may be disclosed, and for what purpose; how long personally identifiable information is retained; the degree to which users can delete or remove information; and the use of passive tracking mechanisms (like cookies) and the purposes for which they are used.

- Organizations must obtain explicit opt-in approval from users before employing passive tracking mechanisms that keep information beyond the user session during which it was collected.

- Organizations must allow users to opt out of the collection and use of personally identifiable information. They also need to describe the consequences of both providing or not providing such information.

- Organizations must not use personally identifiable health information for any purpose outside of what has been disclosed without first obtaining additional opt-in approval.

- Organizations must hold any third party to whom they give access to such data to the same policies that they disclose to users.

- Organizations must do annual security audits to guard against unauthorized access to personal health information.

Adequate assurances of privacy protection are a basic requirement of all Ix applications. All clinics, hospitals, and health plans are encouraged to apply for accreditation for their Web sites or partner with previously accredited health Web sites to deliver information prescriptions to their members and patients.

Information Therapy and the Corporate Practice of Medicine

If the prescription of information to a patient is considered a part of the patient's therapy, it could be considered, under the medical practice acts, something that must be done directly by a professional licensed to practice medicine. A restrictive interpretation of these laws could prevent corporations and nonlicensed persons from providing information prescriptions based on medical information about an individual.

Medical practice acts, enacted in every state in the U.S., set out the qualifications needed to obtain a license to practice medicine and require that no person practice medicine without one. While few states explicitly prohibit corporations from practicing medicine, courts in many jurisdictions have held that because of its nonpersonal nature, a corporation cannot meet the qualifications of the licensure stature and therefore may not practice medicine. This legal doctrine of corporate practice of medicine prohibition has been applied quite differently from state to state.[7]

While concerns about these potential restrictions exist, they are lessened by a number of factors.

- Hospitals and other organizations licensed to provide care have been generally exempted by the courts from the corporate practice prohibitions.[8]

- The rapid proliferation of managed care organizations, for-profit hospitals, specialty medical centers, and other for-profit and not-for-profit organizations has been little affected by the doctrine.

- The protections of freedom of speech under the First Amendment to the U.S. Constitution are broadly interpreted and may broadly apply to information prescriptions.

Still, a legal review of these issues is prudent before pursuing a course of system-prescribed information therapy. In truth, a review of all legal issues pertaining to the prescription of information to patients is prudent.

An Information Therapy Assessment for Clinics

Part 1. Clinic Overview (to be completed by clinic manager or lead physician)

The purpose of the clinic overview is to establish a basic understanding of the staff, their daily interaction with patients, and their awareness of information therapy.

Level of Awareness

- Has anyone been assigned to learn about information therapy?
- Has the board or partnership been briefed on information therapy?
- Have the clinicians been briefed?

Summary of the Practice

- Staff
  - Number of individual and FTE physicians practicing
  - Specialties involved
  - Number of FTE nonphysician clinicians practicing
- Patient load
  - Office visits scheduled per physician per hour (break out by type)
  - Average number of visits scheduled per hour per clinician
  - Average number of patients seen per day (break out by type)
  - Average number of physician and nurse phone calls per clinic visit
- Patient wait times
  - Average patient wait time in lobby (total and after scheduled time)
  - Average patient wait time in exam room
  - Average patient time in clinic overall

Part 2. Physician, Nurse, and Staff Interviews

The purpose of the interviews is to gain clinician and staff insights into the needs and opportunities to improve care through information therapy. Results should be presented grouped by physician, nurse, or other professional. While interview questions may differ, they should provide information similar to that provided below:

- An estimate of how much time is now spent on patient education inside the clinical visit

- A list of clinical situations that account for a significant amount of the patient education time

- A list of clinical situations in which additional patient education and self-management skill building seems to be needed

- A list of preventive measures for which periodic reminders to the patient would be important and helpful

- An assessment of the relative need of patient information for each of the following: self-care; self-triage; visit preparation; visit follow-up and shared decision making; self-management of chronic disease; and end-of-life care information for patients and their families

- Clinician assessment of the reliability of codes used for diagnosis and billing and a description of who does and reviews the coding

- Overall willingness of the clinician to participate in a pilot project to test the use of information prescriptions to patients

- A prioritized list of physician concerns about sending information prescriptions to patients: (e-mail overload, quality of information, privacy, liability, etc.)

- Clinician attitudes and expectations regarding the implementation of computer and wireless technology into their practice

- Specific clinician willingness to use a PDA or tablet PC during clinic visits as part of a pilot project

Part 3. Technical Assessment

The purpose of the technology assessment is to determine what coding and technology infrastructure is in place or planned that might be used within an Ix program. The assessment would be completed by a survey among those responsible for the technology of the clinic.

Coding Systems and Clinical Languages Currently in Use

Rate how precisely the codes are used. Code accuracy helps ensure the precision of Ix prescriptions.

Code/Language	Not used	Inaccurate	Sometimes accurate but needs improvement	Highly accurate
ICD-9				
ICD-10				
CPT®-4				
SNOMED®				
NDC				
Others				

Computer Applications

Indicate the clinic's current status and long-term plans with respect to each area listed below.

Area of Computer Use	Now	Within 1 year	Within 3 years
Billing and accounting by computer			
Schedule keeping by computer			
Computers in physician offices			
Computers in exam rooms			
Computers available for patient use			
% of computers that are networked			
% of computers that have Internet access			
Prescription ordering by computer			
Medical test ordering by computer			
Clinical referral by computer			
Surgery scheduling by computer			
Use of EMR			
Wireless application—prescription ordering			
Wireless application—lab test ordering			
Wireless application—EMR entry			

Part 4: Patient Survey

The fourth element of the assessment is an in-clinic survey of patients to determine both the average patient mix and the patient readiness of Ix applications. The information can be gathered both before and after a clinic visit to take advantage of waiting room time and allow for fresh observations from the clinical encounter.

From Previsit Data Collected in the Waiting Room

- Average age

- Average education level of a visiting patient

- Reasons for visit (selection from a list plus write-ins). For example, percent of visits for:

  - Preventive care

  - Acute health problems

  - Chronic illness management

  - Pediatric patients

  - Patients expecting decisions about surgery, medication, or medical tests

- Timing of visit. Percent of visits that are:

  - Walk-ins

  - "Same day"

  - Scheduled at least one day in advance

- Internet connectivity of patients. Percent of patients:

  - With Internet access

  - With e-mail

  - Who looked for information on the Internet for the health problem they were seeing the doctor for that day

  - Who would value getting informative e-mails from physician

From Postvisit Data Collected Before the Patient Leaves the Clinic

- Clinic visit outcomes

  - Average patient time in clinic (not counting survey time)

  - Percent of visits needing follow-up visit

  - Percent of visits resulting in decision to do medical tests (lab, X-ray, or other)

  - Percent of visits resulting in decisions to proceed to surgery

  - Percent of visits resulting in medication prescriptions (plus number of prescriptions)

- Patient education and understanding

  - Average minutes per visit spent on informing or educating patient (patient estimate)

  - Patient ability to name diagnosis

  - Patient listing of home treatment recommendations

  - Patient listing of treatment plan

  - Patient desire for additional information

Notes

Chapter 2: Four Drivers of Health Care Change

1. Regina E. Herzlinger, *Market-Driven Health Care: Who Wins, Who Loses in the Transformation of America's Largest Service Industry* (Reading, Mass.: Perseus Books, 1997), 3-84.

2. Institute for the Future, *Health and Health Care 2010: The Forecast, The Challenge* (San Francisco: Jossey-Bass Publishers, 2000), 3.

3. Elaine M. Kryouz et al., *Catch the First Wave: Twenty-First Century Health Care Consumers* (Institute for the Future, 1998), 5-6.

4. Arthur Andersen LLP and the Health Forum, *Leadership for a Healthy Twenty-First Century: Creating Value Through Relationships* (1999), as cited in Michael Herrick and Andrew Patterson, "Healthcare Trends—The Big Picture," *Journal of AHIMA* (May 2000). Available at: www.ahima.org/journal/features/feature.0005.1.html (accessed March 2002).

5. Dan Vergano, "The Operation You Get Often Depends on Where You Live," *USA Today*, 19 September 2000, final edition.

6. Dartmouth Medical School, Center for the Evaluative Clinical Sciences, *The Dartmouth Atlas of Health Care, 1999*, The Dartmouth Atlas of Health Care in the United States, eds. John E. Wennberg and Megan McAndrew Cooper (Chicago: American Hospital Association Press, 1999), 167-174.

7. Dartmouth Medical School, *Dartmouth Atlas*.

8. Vergano, "The Operation You Get."

9. David L. Sackett et al., *Evidence-Based Medicine: How to Practice and Teach EBM*, 2nd ed. (Edinburgh: Churchill Livingstone, 2000), 1.

10. National Committee on Quality Assurance, "Beta Blocker Treatment After a Heart Attack," State of Managed Care Quality, 2001. Available at: www.ncqa.org/somc2001/beta_bl/somc_2001_bbh.html (accessed March 2002).

11. A 2000 study done as part of the Pew Internet and American Life Project found that:

> Fifty-two million adult Americans—55% of the Internet-user population—have turned to Internet sources to seek health information. . . . In a comparative sense, more Internet users have sought medical information on the Web than have shopped

online (47% of Internet users have done that), looked up stock quotes (44% of Internet users have done that), or checked sports scores (36% of Internet users have done that). Twenty-nine percent of health seekers, or about 15 million people, go online to look for medical information about once a week and 30% go online once per month. Less-healthy people are more likely to seek such information frequently—32% of those who say they are in less than excellent health go online once per week, compared to 23% of those who say they are in "excellent" health. On a typical day online, about 6% of Internet users are seeking health and medical information. That is more than 5 1/2 million Americans.

Susannah Fox and Lee Rainie, "The Online Health Care Revolution: How the Web Helps Americans Take Better Care of Themselves," Pew Internet and American Life Project: Online Life Report (2000). Available at: http://www.pewinternet.org/reports/index.asp (accessed March 2002).

12. "The Chi Machine," Chi Guide to Better Health [Online]. Available at: http://www.something4u.com/chi/chi.htm (accessed March 2002).

13. "The FIR Hot House Health Builder," Chi Guide to Better Health [Online]. Available at: http://www.something4u.com/chi/fir.htm (accessed March 2002).

14. "Internal Cleansing Dynamics, Inc." Available at: http://store.enempo.com. (accessed March 2002).

15. "Dr. Hulda Clark: The Real Cause of HIV/AIDS." Available at: http://www.drclark.net/hiv/cause_hiv.htm (accessed March 2002).

16. "Dr. Clark's New 21 Day Program for Advanced Cancers." Available at: http://www.drclark.net/info/21days.htm (accessed March 2002).

17. "ADD-ADHD Depression Cure." Available at: http://www.all-organic-food.com/add-adhd.htm (accessed March 2002).

18. RAND Health, "Proceed with Caution: A Report on the Quality of Health Information on the Internet" (California HealthCare Foundation, May 2001).

19. Gretchen K. Berland et al., "Health Information on the Internet: Accessibility, Quality, and Readability in English and Spanish," *Journal of the American Medical Association*, 285, no. 20 (2001): 2620.

20. Childhood Asthma Management Program Research Group, "Long-Term Effects of Budesonide or Nedocromil in Children with Asthma," *New England Journal of Medicine* 343, no. 15 (2000): 1054-1063; Lone Agertoft and Soren Pedersen, "Effect of Long-Term Treatment with Inhaled Budesonide on Adult Height in Children with Asthma," *New England Journal of Medicine* 343, no. 15 (2000): 1064-1069.

21. Committee on Quality of Health Care in America, Institute of Medicine, *To Err is Human: Building a Safer Health System,* eds. Linda T. Kohn, Janet Corrigan, and Molla S. Donaldson (Washington, D.C.: National Academy Press, 2000), 31.

22. Committee on Quality of Health Care in America, Institute of Medicine. *Crossing the Quality Chasm: A New Health System for the Twenty-First Century* (Washington, D.C.: National Academy Press, 2001), 1.

23. Donald Berwick, "Escape Fire" (paper presented at the Eleventh Annual National Forum on Quality Improvement in Health Care, New Orleans, December 1999).

24. The Committee on Quality of Health Care in America (*Crossing the Quality Chasm,* 61-62) has proposed a set of new ideas to guide the reshaping of the health care system:

NEW RULES TO REDESIGN AND IMPROVE CARE

Private and public purchasers, health care organizations, clinicians, and patients should work together to redesign health care processes in accordance with the following rules:

1. **Care based on continuous healing relationships.** Patients should receive care whenever they need it and in many forms, not just face-to-face visits. This rule implies that the health care system should be responsive at all times (24 hours a day, every day) and that access to care should be provided over the Internet, by telephone, and by other means in addition to face-to-face visits.

2. **Customization based on patient needs and values.** The system of care should be designed to meet the most common types of needs, but have the capability to respond to individual patient choices and preferences.

3. **The patient as the source of control.** Patients should be given the necessary information and the opportunity to exercise the degree of control they choose over health care decisions that affect them. The health system should be able to accommodate differences in patient preferences and encourage shared decision-making.

4. **Shared knowledge and the free flow of information.** Patients should have unfettered access to their own medical information and to clinical knowledge. Clinicians and patients should communicate effectively and share information.

5. **Evidence-based decision-making.** Patients should receive care based on the best available scientific knowledge. Care should not vary illogically from clinician to clinician or from place to place.

6. **Safety as a system property**. Patients should be safe from injury caused by the care system. Reducing risk and ensuring safety require greater attention to systems that help prevent and mitigate errors.

7. **The need for transparency**. The health care system should make information available to patients and their families that allows them to make informed decisions when selecting a health plan, hospital, or clinical practice, or when choosing among alternative treatments. This should include information describing the system's performance on safety, evidence-based practice, and patient satisfaction.

8. **Anticipation of needs**. The health system should anticipate patient needs, rather than simply reacting to events.

9. **Continuous decrease in waste**. The health system should not waste resources or patient time.

10. **Cooperation among clinicians**. Clinicians and institutions should actively collaborate and communicate to ensure an appropriate exchange of information and coordination of care.

Reprinted with permission, courtesy of the National Academy Press.

Chapter 3: Prescribing Information

1. "Bunion Removal," MEDLINEplus Medical Encyclopedia [Online]. Available at: www.nlm.nih.gov/medlineplus/ency/article/002962.htm (accessed March 2002).

2. "Magnetic Insoles: Secret to Natural Foot Pain Relief," Magnetic Ideas, Inc. Available at: www.magneticideas.com/footinsoles.htm (accessed March 2002).

3. Amilcare Gentili et al., "Hallux Valgus: Pre- and Postoperative Radiographic Evaluation," *Radiologic Society of North America Electronic Journal* 2 (1998). Available at: http://ej.rsna.org/ej2/ej.htm (accessed March 2002).

4. Frank Davidoff et al., "Evidence-Based Medicine," *British Medical Journal* 310 (29 April 1995): 1085.

5. Ibid., 1085.

6. William Rosenberg and Anna Donald, "Evidence-Based Medicine: An Approach to Clinical Problem-Solving," *British Medical Journal* 310 (29 April 1995): 1122-1126.

7. The Cochrane Collaboration is an international organization that aims to help people make well-informed decisions about health care by preparing, maintaining, and ensuring the accessibility of systematic reviews of the effects of health care interventions. Learn more about the work of the Cochrane Collaboration at www.cochrane.org.

8. The Agency for Healthcare Research and Quality (AHRQ) sponsors and conducts research that provides evidence-based information on health care outcomes; quality; and cost, use, and access. The information helps health care decision makers—patients, clinicians, health system leaders, purchasers, and policy makers—make more informed decisions and improve the quality of health care services. Learn more about the AHRQ at www.ahrq.gov.

9. Sackett et al., *How to Practice and Teach EBM*, 1.

10. David L. Sackett et al., "Evidence-Based Medicine: What It Is and What It Isn't," *British Medical Journal* 312 (13 January 1996): 71-72.

11. U.S. Preventive Services Task Force, *Guide to Clinical Preventive Services*, 2nd ed. (Baltimore: Williams & Wilkins, 1996), 862.

12. Dartmouth Medical School, *Dartmouth Atlas*.

13. "The ABCs of Melanoma," Healthwise® Knowledgebase (Boise, Idaho: Healthwise, Incorporated, 2002). Reprinted with permission of Healthwise, Incorporated.

Chapter 4: Physician-Prescribed Information Therapy

1. Milt Freudenheim, "In a Shift, an HMO Rewards Doctors for Quality Care," *New York Times*, 11 July 2001, late edition.

2. Charles H. Braddock III et al., "Informed Decision Making in Outpatient Practice: Time to Get Back to Basics," *Journal of the American Medical Association* 282, no. 24 (1999): 2313-2320.

3. Committee on Quality of Health Care in America, *Crossing the Quality Chasm*, 166.

Chapter 5: System-Prescribed Information Therapy

1. *Mosby's Medical, Nursing, & Allied Health Dictionary*, 5th ed., revision ed. Kenneth N. Anderson (St. Louis: Mosby-Year Book, Inc., 1998), 1534.

2. Berland et al., "Health Information on the Internet."

3. Braddock et al., "Informed Decision Making in Outpatient Practice."

4. M. W. Kreuter, V. J. Strecher, and B. Glassman, "One Size Does Not Fit All: The Case for Tailoring Print Materials," *Annals of Behavioral Medicine* 21, no. 4 (1999): 276-283.

5. ICD-9-CM, *Millennium Edition, International Classification of Diseases, 9th Revision, Clinical Modification, 6th Edition, 2002* (Los Angeles: Practice Management Information Corporation, 2001).

6. *Current Procedural Terminology* (CPT®), 2002 (Chicago: American Medical Association, 2001).

7. Available at: www.snomed.org (accessed March 2002).

8. Available at: www.hl7.org (accessed March 2002).

9. Mark Stega et al., *Context Management ("CCOW") Specification, Subject Data Definitions, Version CM-1.3* (Ann Arbor: Health Level 7).

Chapter 6: Consumer-Prescribed Information Therapy

1. Oregon Health Sciences University, Final Grant Report, Healthwise Evaluation Project, Robert Wood Johnson Foundation Grant ID# 027929 (May 1, 1996, to November 30, 1999).

2. Ibid.

3. Blue Cross of Idaho 1996-1997 claims analysis.

4. Oregon Health Sciences University Physician Interviews (1997).

5. Oregon Health Sciences University, Final Grant Report.

Chapter 7: Business Opportunities in Information Therapy

1. Edward H. Wagner et al., "The Effect of a Shared Decisionmaking Program on Rates of Surgery for Benign Prostatic Hyperplasia: Pilot Results," *Medical Care* 33, no. 8 (1995): 765-70.

2. Angelique M. van den Belt et al., "Fixed Dose Subcutaneous Low Molecular Weight Heparins Versus Adjusted Dose Unfractionated Heparin for Venous Thromboembolism (Cochrane Review)," *The Cochrane Library*, 1 (Oxford: Update Software, 2002).

3. Cornerstone Communications Group, "Analysis of American Nurses Association Staffing Survey" (American Nurses Association, February 2001). Available at: www.ana.org/surveys (accessed March 2002).

4. As cited in First Consulting Group, "E-Encounters," eHealth Report for the California HealthCare Foundation (November 2001). Available at: admin.chcf.org/documents/ehealth/EEncounters.pdf (accessed March 2002).

5. Pharmaceutical Care Management Association, "How Many Americans Are Served by PBMs?" [Online]. Available at: www.pcmanet.org/home.html (accessed March 2002).

6. Express Scripts, "Direct-to Consumer Advertising Proves Its Power to Influence Prescription Drug Consumption," 2000: *Top Developments on the Pharmaceutical Landscape* [Online]. Available at: www.express-scripts.com (accessed March 2002).

7. Michael S. Wilkes, Robert A. Bell, and Richard L. Kravitz, "Direct-to-Consumer Prescription Drug Advertising: Trends, Impact, and Implications," *Health Affairs* 19, no. 2 (2000): 110-28.

8. Kaiser Family Foundation, press release, "Understanding the Effects of Direct-to-Consumer Prescription Drug Advertising, 2001" (21 November 2001).

9. Express Scripts, "Direct-to-Consumer Advertising."

10. Disease Management Association of America, "Definition of Disease Management" [Online]. Available at: www.dmaa.org (accessed March 2002).

11. "AHRQ Profile: Quality Research for Quality Health Care." Available at: www.ahrq.gov (accessed March 2002).

12. Wendy Levinson et al., "Physician-Patient Communication: The Relationship with Malpractice Claims among Primary Care Physicians and Surgeons," *Journal of the American Medical Association* 227, no. 7 (1997): 553.

13. Levinson et al., "Physician-Patient Communication," 553.

14. The *JAMA* article by Levinson et al. uncovers other fascinating information about physicians who are "no-claims." One tidbit is that "no-claims physicians used humor more often and laughed more." We thought you'd like to know.

Chapter 8: Health Care in an Information Therapy Future

1. Committee on Quality of Healthcare in America, *Crossing the Quality Chasm*, 181.

2. Ibid.

3. Go to www.ehealthinitiative.org to learn more about eHI and its efforts to restructure medical reimbursement.

4. Prepared by Gregory R. Riley, Legal Research Assistant, The Pennsylvania State University, The Dickinson School of Law, June 2001.

5. "What Is Contract Law?" Arizona Bar Foundation. Available at: www.lawforkids.org/QA/other/other98.cfm (accessed March 2002).

6. Robert D. Orr et al., "The Use of the Hippocratic Oath: A Review of Twentieth-Century Practice and a Content Analysis of Oaths Administered in Medical Schools in the U.S. and Canada in 1993," *Journal of Clinical Ethics* 8, no. 4 (1997): 377-88.

7. Although many medical schools today used modernized versions of the Hippocratic oath, their central promises are those of the traditional version:

> I SWEAR by Apollo the physician, AEsculapius, and Health, and All-heal, and all the gods and goddesses, that, according to my ability and judgement, I will keep this Oath and this stipulation.

> TO RECKON him who taught me this Art equally dear to me as my parents, to share my substance with him, and relieve his necessities if required; to look up his offspring in the same footing as my own brothers, and to teach them this art, if they shall wish to learn it, without fee or stipulation; and that by precept, lecture, and every other mode of instruction, I will impart a knowledge of the Art to my own sons, and those of my teachers, and to disciples bound by a stipulation and oath according the law of medicine, but to none others.

> I WILL FOLLOW that system of regimen which, according to my ability and judgment, I consider for the benefit of my patients, and abstain from whatever is deleterious and mischievous. I will give no deadly medicine to any one if asked, nor suggest any such counsel; and in like manner I will not give a woman a pessary to produce abortion.

> WITH PURITY AND WITH HOLINESS I will pass my life and practice my Art. I will not cut persons laboring under the stone, but will leave this to be done by men who are practitioners of this work. Into whatever houses I enter, I will go into them for the benefit of the sick, and will abstain from every voluntary act of mischief and corruption; and, further from the seduction of females or males, of freemen and slaves.

> WHATEVER, IN CONNECTION with my professional practice or not, in connection with it, I see or hear, in the life of men, which ought not to be spoken of abroad, I will not divulge, as reckoning that all such should be kept secret.

> WHILE I CONTINUE to keep this Oath unviolated, may it be granted to me to enjoy life and the practice of the art, respected by all men, in all times! But should I trespass and violate this Oath, may the reverse be my lot!

8. The time has come, Dr. Greene says, "to put [the Hippocratic] oath on a shelf of honor in medical history, to be replaced not by an updated version, but by a fundamentally new oath to launch us into the future of health." Below is the Millennium Health Oath he proposes.

> I SWEAR by Health, and by the global human community, and by Earth our planet that, according to my ability and judgment, I will keep this Oath and will reckon those who benefit from the Art of Medicine dear to me. I will teach them this Art, if they shall wish to learn it. And by precept, lecture, and every other mode of instruction, I will impart knowledge of Health to them.

> In whatever I say or do I will follow the course that, according to my ability and judgment, I consider for the benefit of their health, and abstain from whatever is deleterious and mischievous. I will deal with people truthfully and without deception, not overreaching the scope of my expertise.

> I will seek always to improve my wisdom, knowledge, and expertise, learning from Science, from other physicians, from nurses, from patients, and from others, in order to deliver the highest quality and most up-to-date care. I will provide also the means for people to evaluate that which I recommend and the means to make their own health decisions with the benefit of my expertise and thoughtful counsel.

> Into whatever homes I enter, I will go into them for the benefit of the people's health. I will practice my art with purity, and make clear any competing benefit, claim, or hindrance that might influence what I say or do. I will abstain from sexual misconduct and from every voluntary act of mischief and corruption; and, further from misleading anyone or seeking hidden financial gain.

> Whatever, in connection with my professional practice or not, I see or hear in the lives of people that ought not to be spoken of abroad, I will not divulge, as reckoning that all such should be kept secret. Whatever health-related personal information I collect I will safeguard it, and use it only for purposes agreed to by the person or demanded by conscience.

> While I continue to keep this Oath unviolated, may it be granted to me to enjoy life and the practice of the art, respected by all people, in all times! But should I trespass and violate this Oath, may the reverse be my lot!

Alan Greene, "Millennium Health Oath Calls Doctors to Practice Medicine in a Whole New Way!" www.drgreene.com.

Appendix A: Legal Issues in Information Therapy

1. American College of Legal Medicine Textbook Committee, *Legal Medicine*, 4th ed. (St. Louis: Mosby, 1998), 260.

2. Ibid., 260-261.

3. Ibid., 261.

4. Ibid., 261-262.

5. Ibid., 123.

6. Ibid., 123.

7. Jeffrey F. Chase-Lubitz, "The Corporate Practice of Medicine Doctrine: An Anachronism in the Modern Health Care Industry," *Vanderbilt Law Review* 40:445 (1987).

8. *Berlin v. Sarah Bush Lincoln Health Center*, 279 Ill. App. 3d 447 (23 Oct 1997).

Index

CPT (Current Procedural Terminology)
   coding, 78, 103, 104, 163
      for reimbursement, 194
Crisis in health care, 13
Crossing the Quality Chasm, 23, 25, 193
   see also Institute of Medicine

D

Dartmouth Atlas of Health Care, 16, 17
   and geography as destiny, 17
   and surgery variations, 16
Decision support
   and disease management, 171
   and information therapy, 43
   and nurse care counselors, 170, 171
   prescriptions, 62
   service companies, 170
Decision-focused information, 3, 28-31
Decisions
   about health behavior, 30
   about quality of care, 31
   direct medical care, 28
   impact of Ix on, 78
   information focused on, 28-31
Definity Health, 151
Destiny Health, 152
Digital bedsides, 158
Direct-to-consumer medication ads, 172
   regulation of, 174
Disease management
   decision-support companies and,
      171
   and health mastery, 178
   and information therapy, 42
Disease management companies, 175
   example of, 177
   goals of, 175
   reimbursement models for, 176
   triggers from, 176
Doctors
   see Physicians
Doctor Goodwell (virtual clinic), 67, 69,
   164
Dot-com collapse, 137

E

Educating patients
   see Patient education
Education, higher, 186
Efficiency
   see Work flow
eHealth Code of Ethics, 38
eHealth Initiative (eHI), 194
Electronic medical record (EMR),
   companies, 167
      documentation for reimbursement,
      193
      examples of use in Ix, 48, 94
      Ix applications for, 168
      triggering information in, 168
E-mail
   and risks to privacy, 217
   use in physician-prescribed Ix, 49,
      51, 53
   use in system-prescribed Ix, 85, 89,
      93, 97, 99
End-of-life care, 43
Errors
   see Medical errors
Ethics of health information
   agencies that regulate, 38, 216
   confidentiality, 216
   disclosure of commercial
      sponsorship, 38
   regulation of quality, 180, 182, 183
   see also Hippocratic oath
E-transaction companies, 170
Evidenced-based information, 3, 31-35,
196
   and validation for reimbursement,
      192
Evidenced-based medicine, 16, 196
   as driver of change, 13, 16-18
   and Cochrane Collaboration, 32
   components of, 32-33
      diagram of, 32
   definition of, 17
   patient values in, 34, 196

Medical errors—continued

Institute of Medicine report, 23
and malpractice, 215
and pharmacy benefit management
companies, 174
prescription errors, 172
reduced by wireless systems,
156-158
Medical guidance systems, 18
Medical languages, structured
in clinics, 223
in intelligent content, 40-41, 103
problems with, 106
Medical law
see Legal issues
Medical malpractice
see Malpractice
Medical outcomes
improved by Ix, 140
Medical review boards
for content, 36
Medical schools, 186
Hippocratic oath in, 198
and shared decision making, 186
Medication orders
as triggers, 94
Medicine
as a science, 16-18
as an art, 16-18
corporate practice of, 218
Memorial Hospital and Health System,
161
Messages to patients, 100
Millennium Health Oath, 199, 235
Mistakes
see Medical errors
Morrison family, 10
information prescriptions for, 48, 84,
92, 96, 120
Moments in care
challenge in focusing on, 119
and clinical qualifiers, 82
and consumer-prescribed Ix, 119
definition of, 46, 79

examples of (for congestive heart
failure), 80-81
identifying, 168
predicting, 76, 78
and reimbursement criteria, 193
and system-prescribed Ix, 77, 79
table, 80-81
Multimedia, 7, 39-40
MyHealthBank, 153

N

National Center for Complementary
and Alternative Medicine, 117
National Committee for Quality
Assurance (NCQA), 146, 181, 216
NDC (National Drug Code), 105, 163
New consumer
as driver of change, 13, 14-16
Baby Boomers as, 14
characteristics of, 14-15
expectations of, 5, 15
physician expectations of, 130-131
New science
see Evidence-based medicine
Nonwired settings, 47, 55, 57-58
Nurses
American Nurses Association
survey, 155
as care counselors, 170, 171
in clinics, 162
in hospitals, 155
patient education and, 162-163
shortage of, 155

O

O.A.S.I.S.: (Online Asperger Syndrome
Information and Support), 127, 128
Opportunities for information therapy,
41-43
see also Business opportunities in Ix
Outcomes, medical
consumer influence on, 195